DATE DUE

THE LIFE OF ILLNESS

SUNY SERIES,
THE BODY IN CULTURE,
HISTORY, AND RELIGION

HOWARD EILBERG-SCHWARTZ, EDITOR

THE LIFE OF ILLNESS

One Woman's Journey

Carol T. Olson

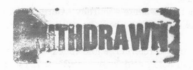

STATE UNIVERSITY OF NEW YORK PRESS

Published by
State University of New York Press, Albany

Printed in the United States of America

For information, address State University of New York
Press, State University Plaza, Albany, N.Y., 12246

Production by Diane Ganeles
Marketing by Dana E. Yanulavich

Library of Congress Cataloging-in-Publication Data

Olson, Carol T., 1951–
    The life of illness : one woman's journey / Carol T. Olson.
        p.   cm. — (SUNY series, the body in culture, history, and
    religion)
    Includes bibliographical references and index.
    ISBN 0-7914-1199-0 (CH : acid-free). — ISBN 0-7914-1200-8 (PB :
acid-free)
    1. Olson, Carol T., 1951–   . 2. Kidneys—Diseases—Patients—
United States—Biography. 3. Hemodialysis. 4. Chronic diseases—
Psychological aspects. I. Title. II. Series.
RC902.O47 1993
362.1'9661'0092—dc20
    [B]   91-33457
                                                           CIP

10 9 8 7 6 5 4 3 2 1

To my Father and Mother
and brothers and sisters
with prayer for all
who keep vigil during illness

CONTENTS

INTRODUCTORY ESSAY: OTHERS

The reader of Carol Olson's thoroughly compelling and deeply stirring text *The Life of Illness* soon learns the importance of a word that acquires many layered and complex significances. This word is "other." The first time other appears in the book it possesses rather innocent meaning. This occurs in the opening pages of Joy's Diary. The "others" were Joy's classmates. The others could do things she could not do. The others left her far behind on the running track. The others could not understand why she was so tired. The others were also those to whom Joy wanted to prove something. And as the readers of her diary we ache for the pain that Joy experiences as a result of her illness and of the seemingly unbridgable abyss, between the self and the others.

On the one hand the illness itself is this abyss, this chasm that separates the ill person from the others. On the other hand, the abyss can also be seen as the relation between self and other. It is this ambiguous abyss that Carol sets out to explore in all its dangerous crevices where death and despair loom, but her journey also offers magical vistas and rich plateaus where we are blessed with understandings. We come to understand that living with illness is also the strange blessing that helps give voice to life and to the meaning of living with others. Sometimes the power of this voice becomes so sonorous that it may leave us, the others, breathless.

Of course, there is always the problem that the others, the healthy ones, may not understand. The medical doctor and psychologist van den Berg provides startling insight into the nature of this possible nonunderstanding. In a rather down-to-earth manner he shows how the room where the ill person spends so much time can open to a world full of wonders and fundamental life experiences. The person who lives with illness is often able to see things and interpret phenomena in ways that seem curious, odd, or strange. From the healthy person's point of view, the ill person seems to sublimate for his or her desires by substituting for normal things that are now out of reach. "If the healthy person states that a patient sublimates, he wishes to say that the sick person by-passes the real values of life and finds solace in poor substitutes" (1980, 73). But van den Berg shows that the healthy person's view demonstrates serious misunderstanding of the relation between wellness and illness in healthy and ill people. He proposes a radical reversal of common sense:

> Who misses more of life, the healthy person, when he throws himself into the avalanche of ever more respect, with an ever more wonderful house, an ever more expensive car and ever further reaching holiday trips, and consequently a frantic drive for money; when he throws himself into this avalanche which bears the dazzling name of 'career'? Or the sick person who makes his room, his windowsill, his window and his view a world full of significant and breathtaking events? Who—now in a completely different sense— is more ill? The illness of the body can be the condition for a soundness of mind which the healthy person misses easily. An existence devoid of sickness lacks the stimulus to live, just as an existence devoid of mental problems degenerates into complete insignificance. Probably there is no better guarantee for a really unhealthy life than perfect health.

We do not need to read Carol's book *The Life of Illness* to know that it would be seriously sacrilegious to talk of the blessings of being ill. And yet, van den Berg is not making light of things that are grave. Rather he forces us to question of what is the meaning of illness and health in our lives. This is also the question that is the thrust in Carol Olson's *The Life of Illness.*

Having known Carol, Joy, Arthur, and their truly heroic mother I never failed to experience a certain "coming to my senses" when I met Joy in the hallways of the university or Arthur in their dialysis room or when I continue to visit Carol and her mother, Mrs. Olson. These encounters always leave me with the experience of having met the other in myself and myself in the other. What is this meaning of the other? How can we experience the other? For this we must first overcome a common but narrow understanding and identification with self. In order to contextualize Carol Olson's use of the notion of other in this text I will briefly discuss some philosophical foundations of Emmanuel Levinas (1969, 1981, 1985).

To be able to understand the meaning of otherness we must overcome an orientation to the world that seems to come naturally to human beings, the attitude of seeing oneself at the center of all things. Every human experiences the taken-for-granted relation of self to the world: I live my life; this is my world in which I live. I am at home in my world. "I live here" means I exist here and I belong here. When I speak or interact with others, I am constantly the subject of my discourse and my actions: I think, I see, I feel, I hear, I understand, I love, I do, I play, I wonder about things. I am involved in projects in the world which define my relation to the world, and which show who I am in the world. I make a meal. I favor certain foods. I enjoy reading a book. I have an opinion about certain people or about what they do. I work at certain things. I am proud about my accomplishments or I feel dissatisfied or unhappy with what I have done or what others do to me. I may go to a movie, to the pub, or to church. The point is, I am the center of my universe. I am my world.

When things go well I may feel "on top of the world." Everything seems just right. The things in the world exist as if they are there just for me. This world is my home, my kingdom. I belong here. But sometimes this experience of the centrality of the "I" can suddenly turn existentially into a crisis, for example, when I suddenly face a serious illness. Now I feel forsaken, shaken. This will be my death. In the awareness of my mortality and of my impending end, my world, my future can shrink into a small circle of despair.

This experience of the primacy of the "I" in my world is neither good nor bad. It is the way human beings may experience the world, know the world, recognize the world as theirs. But of course this is not the whole of human experience. The human being is not alone. Some people may prize aloneness, independence, separateness; others may suffer from loneliness and alienation from others. Yet in these experiences the felt absence or presence of others is already implicit. In the world we experience the other person. There are other people who live beside me. There are others whom I encounter in the world. The question is: How do the others appear to me? Are they there simply for me, as parts of my larger world? Are the others only important for me in so far that they add to or subtract from my world? Are the others just there as objects for the satisfaction of my wants and needs: to be used, manipulated, made available by me and to me?

I do not really experience the subjectivity of the other until I am able to overcome the centeredness of my self in the world. The fascinating fact is that my possibility of the experience of the otherness of other, resides in my experience of the vulnerability of the other. It is when I see that the other is a person who can be hurt, distressed, pained, suffering, anguished, weak, in grief, or in despair that I may be opened to the essential being of the other. The vulnerability of the other is the weak spot in the armor of the self-centered world. I see a person who is hurt or who is in agony and, temporarily at least, I forget my present preoccupations. No longer am I driven by my personal agenda. For the moment I am just there for this child, man, or woman. With this recognition of the other comes the possibility of acting for the sake of the other. And so when a person is ill and I actually "see" this person in his or her vulnerability then I am temporarily lifted over the boundary-chasm of self-centeredness that separates me from experiencing the other as other. This then, says Levinas, is the experience of unselfishness, of responsibility by and for the other. In order to understand this experience of responsibility Levinas develops the phenomenology of the face.

When someone turns to me I primarily experience the face of the other. Here is someone who looks me in the eyes. And in this face I experience the immediate presence of someone other. Levinas shows us that this meeting has a peculiar human ethical structure—as in what may happen when we meet a playing child in the street who greets and smiles at us. The very moment that we turn to this uplifted face we are addressed in our fundamental responsibility.

For Levinas the ethical is always in the concrete, in the situation in which the other bursts upon my world. Intersubjectivity is not something that I create or give shape to through some kind of dialogic encounter. Rather, the Other is given to me as an ethical event in the confrontative recognition of the face—the face that I recognize as my responsibility for the other. And this ethical situation cannot be theorized, cannot be conceptually understood as situation in its contingency. Levinas does not think of intersubjectivity in a methodological, ontological, or epistemological way, but rather as a kind of moral experience that happens to you. "Face and discourse are tied. The face speaks. It speaks, it is in this that it renders possible and begins all discourse. . . it is discourse and, more exactly, response or responsibility which is this authentic relationship" (Levinas 1985, 87).

Many parents have experienced the situation of sitting at the bedside of their sick child. After some innocent symptoms the child has suddenly become seriously ill. And now I see my child suffering with a high fever and with a strange vacant expression in the eyes. This child is more than just a worry that will soon pass. Although the child is totally passive, making no demands on me, it is as if my world is nevertheless pressuring me to forget everything that hitherto seemed important. The whole world is simply reduced to this child in this sickroom. The child's suffering has become my suffering. If only I could take the place of my child! I know that I am responsible for this sick child even though I am not the cause of this suffering. I cannot help but experience my responsibility for this child, for this other person. As Carol Olson shows us, responsibility is being there as "one for the other."

This is, I believe, how Carol Olson wants us to begin to reflect with her on the significance of the other in the experience of illness. I would use the word 'heteronomy' to describe something that goes beyond the self-centered principle of autonomy, independence. Heteronomy is the other side of autonomy: it means to be claimed or dependent on something that comes from the outside. The heteronomy of responsibility is at the heart of my relation to my child, it is the call the other makes on my personal responsibility. My responsibility has made me dependent on the other to whom I stand in a nursing or pedagogical relation. Thus, one could speak of the heteronomy of the vocation of nursing, the heteronomy of pedagogy, of ministering, of medical care.

In this book chapters are titled: "One against the other searches for the other." "One with the other." "One for the other." "One by the other." "One without the other." It is by means of these provocative phrases that Carol Olson explores many forms of the substitutive heteronomy of responsibility: the nurse, the minister, the doctor, the mother, the patient. All are called to their ethical encounter with the other.

                                        Max van Manen

ACKNOWLEDGMENTS

To my Mother, for her love and encouragement, her faith and faithfulness, and her strength and gentleness, always a source of life for me. Her very practical help in bringing about improvements in dialysis life and in the research writing and reading of the manuscript are gratefully acknowledged.

To Max and Judith van Manen, for their understanding friendship and help. I thank Max van Manen, Professor of Education at the University of Alberta, for his commitment of very much time, effort, knowledge and talent to the entire project of research writing and publication.

To Priscilla Ross, for her cordial advice and assistance regarding publication. To Diane Ganeles, for her thorough work as production editor.

To Ted Aoki, Professor Emeritus and former Chairman of the Department of Secondary Education at the University of Alberta, for journeying with me in this research of illness; and to Howard Eilberg-Schwartz, Professor of Religious Studies at Stanford University; Maggie Neal, Professor at the University of Baltimore School of Nursing; Vangie Bergum, Professor of Nursing at the University of Alberta; and Marilyn Ray, Eminent Scholar, Christine E. Lynn Chair in Nursing, Florida Atlantic University, for their helpful and supportive reviews of the manuscript.

To the chaplain, the doctor, the nurse, and my mother, whom I interviewed, for their willingness to participate insightfully in the research of illness. To the medical professionals and hospital workers, blood donors and the Canadian Red Cross, Medicare, and dialysis researchers, who have helped me live to write this book.

To Hector F. De Luca, Steenbock Research Professor and Chairman of the Department of Biochemistry of the University of Wisconsin-Madison, and his co-workers, for the development of the kidney active form of vitamin D, which has given bone life to my family on dialysis.

To all who have shared with me the friendship of kind and encouraging conversations and written communications, and to the readers of this book, for their openness to a new author.

INTRODUCTION

Illness in My Family

The following question dwells in my life: "Can we understand the life of illness?" The question emerged in childhood, when my oldest brother, Eddie, and my baby sister, Grace, died of kidney failure and related causes. When I was ten years old, my mother told me I had kidney failure, too. During my teen years my younger sisters, Joy and Crystal, and I were frequently in hospital as the disease progressed. Crystal died when I was in high school. The following year, 1969, my older brother Arthur experienced the sudden collapse of his kidneys with Hong Kong flu and began dialysis on the artifical kidney machine. Joy and I started dialysis two years later. Our years on dialysis together ended when Joy and Arthur died in 1983. My father had died from a heart attack in 1979. Yet the meaning of their lives is not primarily that they died but how they lived.

When I was a child, my father told me that love is like duty, though freely given. My parents lived this love in our home. My father was a minister of the Evangelical Lutheran Church in Canada, serving congregations in Prince Rupert in British Columbia, Moose Jaw in Saskatchewan, and Edmonton in Alberta before becoming Director of the Canadian Lutheran Evangelistic Movement and first President and Director for the World Mission Prayer League (Canada) in 1972. He was also a radio pastor for many years. "Although the work of the church always had priority," Mother once wrote, "he was deeply devoted and dedicated to his family." My father supported us in many ways: he drove

1

Joy and me to and from high school because we could not walk the distance; he carried Joy up the stairs of a university building so she could attend classes there; he prepared Arthur's machine for dialysis while Arthur was suffering from a debilitating bone disease and loss of eyesight. As we needed such physical support, so we needed the spiritual support of his uncompromising faith: he trusted God to provide a way for us each day. When my father's itinerary took him away from home, my mother took over many responsibilities, including driving. She learned to drive at the age of fifty! Typically, Mother was busy with household tasks and yard-work, doctoring and nursing, and her heart was before God in prayer for her family, sustaining us through the day or night.

Mother had been a high school teacher and principal before her marriage, and there was system in our home. As children, with Mother as our teacher, we each practised the piano thirty minutes a day. Arthur accompanied congregational singing, soloists, and wedding processions on piano or organ and became concert master of the All City Junior High School Orchestra. The family was not surprised, therefore, when he chose to teach music for his life's work. To prepare himself, he earned his Bachelor's degree in Secondary Education, with a major in music and minor in political science; followed by his Master's degree in Music Education, teaching orchestra in the Music Education Laboratory at the University of Alberta.

Arthur was dedicated to *public* education, strongly believing that he should provide the opportunity for each child to achieve his full potential. Because a child can learn to love good music and "nothing succeeds like success," his music program was performance-oriented: every child in the school performed in a concert at least twice during the year. More than one hundred children volunteered their noon hours for choir practice. Some of these children gave other free time for recorder band and bell choir practice. Primary children had choral sol-fa and instrumental Orff experience. Following concert performances, Arthur never claimed the applause;

he always faced the children. They had given their all for music and for him. He was their teacher; and the applause belonged to them.

Music became a community project as Arthur directed Webber's operetta, *Joseph's Amazing Technicolor Dreamcoat*, then Gilbert and Sullivan's *H.M.S. Pinafore*. Arthur had begun to work with the children on Humperdinck's *Hansel and Gretel* with its beautiful evening prayer, "When At Night I Go To Sleep," when he died suddenly.

As children, we were accustomed to kneeling at the bedside for our evening prayers with Mother leading us. Father led morning devotions, followed by family singing of a morning prayer and The Lord's Prayer. As soon as we could read, we took turns leading supper devotions and choosing a hymn for the family to sing. We loved this responsibility and surmise that Joy, almost three years younger than I, taught herself to read because she wanted her turn! Because of this ability, she was promoted from kindergarten to grade two.

Joy's love of reading deepened through the years to an author's sensitive appreciation for words. When she was in high school, Joy wrote her diary which begins this book. The family was not surprised when she chose to teach reading and language for her life's work. To prepare herself, she earned her Bachelor's degree in Elementary Education in reading at the University of Alberta and taught remedial reading in a city school. She returned for her Master's degree in Elementary Education in language. With "pedagogic love" Joy transformed her large office, the Reading Clinic for the Learning Disabled in the Department of Educational Psychology, into a child-friendly learning space. All she needed were some knickknacks from home, a jug of juice and her presence as teacher. Joy also worked with student teachers in her office and was a faculty consultant for student teachers in city schools. She had just completed developing a course project for Education students studying English as a Second Language, when she died suddenly. How could Arthur and Joy accomplish so much with so little time and energy? Their secret belongs to God.

Arthur, Joy, and I began independent dialysis in 1976 in a family ward with the assistance of one or two helpers and home dialysis technicians. At home, we discussed our medical concerns around the kitchen table, deferring to Arthur's opinion regarding our medical care. His keen medical insight was honed when he balanced blood serum levels of calcium and phosphate with minute quantities of the kidney-activated form of vitamin D provided by an American researcher in biochemistry, Dr. H.F. De Luca, to mineralize bone and walk again. Beginning with thirty percent bone, Arthur was walking in four months and moving freely in eight months. He was the first person in the world to do so.

Introducing My Work

When tiny human kidneys collapse, their work in our bodies becomes visible in our lives as the artifical kidney machine. The technology of dialysis has advanced to the point where individual needs on dialysis are programmed as variables for the computerized monitor. This technology revitalized my life in the winter of 1991 when I could no longer eat because of a severe reaction to another technology, a stomach medication.

Medical technology gives me life. But medical technology has no life—no soul that suffers pain and abounds in hope. And so technology is mute about the pain it requires of us, the hope it inspires in us, the life it gives us. The silence of technology becomes a question within us: "What is life that technology is not sufficient for life?" This question turns us to what is beyond us, to God, and the search for what is good in the re-search of daily life.

How could I research the life of illness in a way that would help understand how one ought to live? Gadamer writes that understanding is action. Therefore, I searched the actions of those who live in illness and with illness to let show their understanding.

In my research I could not theorize myself out of the pain and the hope, the life of illness. I stand in illness in my research, as in my life, before God, one of the world in pain and hope. I want to live in understanding. I want to learn how one ought to live through illness, even through the grief of pain and death. Finding the themes of pain and hope requires reflection: thinking from the heart of mute experience to come to the heart of the written word. Literary texts show the silence of illness through the voice of the individual, reverberating with the heart of one's experience, shared by all. Still, the words of the shared understanding—themes, are not easily articulated. Whereas the literary author lets the themes rest in the writing, the researcher searches for the words of the themes as they are shown through the writing. Explanation would stop the question, "How ought we to live?" but themes reveal possibilities for living in this question until the themes themselves become open to deeper understanding.

The deepest understanding this research has yielded is a quiet saying: the good of illness is love. From love springs thought that is full of care and care that is full of thought. In illness, there is no life in us other than the love of God for us. There is no life for us other than the love of family, friends, and community; and our love for them. Some live to love the multitude, like Mother Teresa. But she began her ministry by loving an individual. When the House for the Dying was not yet, Mother Teresa felt compassion for a dying beggar on a street of Calcutta. She carried him to her lodging, laid him on her bed, cleaned him up, and nursed him back to health. He asked nothing of her but his need took all she was and had. He gave Mother Teresa her life's work, he became her first helper.

How ought we to live during illness? Though this book is written, the question is new each morning. The good of understanding, the action of love—God's love, is you.

CHAPTER 1

EPIGRAPH FOR JOY

Then bear a joy where joy is not,
Go, speak a kindly word in love.

—F. G. Lee

Joy's Diary

I was born on May 14, 1954, the fourth child in a family of six. My mother wanted to name me Joanne. With my birth, my parents were blessed with two sons and two daughters. My father wanted to name me Joy as befitted the occasion. My parents decided to christen me Joy Margaret.

By the time I was ten years old, my eldest brother, Eddie, had died from kidney failure; my baby sister, Grace Evangeline, had died from probable kidney failure, and my older sister, Carol, had had a kidney biopsy which resulted in a diagnosis of kidney failure.

My own kidney failure showed itself in the form of nephrosis when I was three. Signs of kidney failure showed up briefly when I was in elementary school, but I was in grade nine before definite signs of kidney failure were evidenced.

In 1964, when I was in grade five, I had scarlatina, a mild form of scarlet fever which left me somewhat weak. Although I was light and agile and could run swiftly, I had no endurance, and my strength in physical activities was short-lived. In volleyball, I could never get the ball over the net on my serve; in basketball, I would tire easily from running, and in baseball, the bat was always too heavy for me. I remember that once I was so proud because I had actually swung and hit the ball. However, the swing was so weak that the pitcher caught the ball immediately and I didn't even make it to first base.

7

Even with the lack of endurance, my goal in grade six was to get a senior athletic award. I was good in broad jump, relay, and in running short distances, and by staying with this type of activity, I made it. But not without a struggle.

There was a big schoolyard track that we had to run around four times in order to get our points. Timing played an important part. We went in teams of four. The job was to alternately jog and walk until the assignment was completed.

I started with the others, but very quickly I dropped to the back of the line. After the first round, I was far behind the others and very tired, but I was determined to see it through. With great effort, I jogged some, then walked some, but by the last lap I only had strength for a short walk. Long after the others had completed their lap, I came walking in—ashamed to know what my time was. I threw myself on the ground. My lungs were aching, my chest was heaving, and there was blood in my throat. The others couldn't understand why I was so tired with such a poor performance. At the time, I didn't think much about it. When grade seven came, though, I was completely excused from all physical education classes.

In 1968, when I was in grade nine, I was to learn the meaning of sorrow and the depths of grief.

Crystal, my younger sister by three years, and I were very close. We did everything together.

Since my father was a minister, church was an important part of our lives. It was very natural for us, when we were small, to play ``church'' on Sunday afternoons. We would go down to the basement to the playroom, which was a room that was filled with all of the essentials for little girls—dolls, cribs, dishes, doll clothes, baby carriages, and books.

After dinner, on Sundays, Crystal and I would march downstairs and dress our dolls in their best attire for 'church'. We then carried all of our dolls up to the main floor. If we were lucky and the living room was unoccupied, the chesterfield became the pews and the piano became the church organ. However, at most times, the steps that led upstairs were the pews and the hallway was our speaking platform.

We lined our dolls up on the steps. I would introduce Crystal as the junior choir director. She would then get up and sing as she directed the 'junior choir', usually made up of six dolls. Finally, I introduced Crystal for a solo, and then Crystal introduced me for a solo. Then it would be time to collect our dolls and head for home.

This was a weekly routine for some time. When company came, Crystal and I would always sit in the same chair. When it came to jelly beans, we would divide the beans color by color; and if it came down to one odd one left, that was bitten in two and shared.

When I had scarlatina, I was weakened; but when Crystal caught the disease from me, she had even more difficulty, and was never really strong after that.

By the time she was in grade four, kidney failure was very evident. At that time, my parents were unaware of the name, but her bones were getting weak, stiff, and painful, and she had difficulty walking. We learned later that she had developed "renal rickets". Because the kidneys were not functioning properly, the parathyroid glands were taking over and secreting a hormone called parathormone which was forcing the calcium out of the bones. The result was that the bones were becoming soft and painful. This was really rickets; only since it was caused by lack of renal or kidney function, it was called renal rickets.

Saturday was the day that we got our allowance. Crystal and I took the orders from the family for candy treats, and then headed for the local candy store. We did this summer and winter and enjoyed the walk.

We would go up the back alley, over a log, and then across a small field called McKernan Park. After crossing two connected streets we were at the local string of stores.

However, the time came when Mom said to me, "Maybe you better go to the store by yourself this time." And that was the last time that Crystal and I made our routine trek together.

I remember when Crystal had to start getting blood transfusions because her hemoglobin was constantly dropping due to kidney failure. This caused a condition of anemia which blood transfusions temporarily relieved by raising the red blood count.

I remember that Carol and I told Crystal that she would just have one small needle, and then the transfusion. How little did I know and understand at that time. Crystal's veins were small and it was hard to get a needle into her. Time and again she was poked for one transfusion. Sometimes her foot even had to be pierced. But she kept her suffering to herself and never spoke of the pain to walk or any other pain she suffered. I never knew what she was going through with low hemoglobin and bone disease until I, too, experienced everything firsthand in my own body.

Carol and I decided to give Crystal a little something everytime she needed a transfusion. One time it was popcorn. Another time it was a troll doll, and once it was a teenage doll.

Mom told me one day, outside on the patio, that Crystal didn't have long to live. I knew she had kidney trouble, but I never expected anything as serious as death. I just looked at Mom and said, "Is it that bad?" But I refused to believe it and blocked it from my mind. It just couldn't happen. Yet in my heart I knew it could.

My prayers confirmed what I knew in my heart to be true, yet denied with my mind. With childlike determination, I told God that Eddie and Grace were taken. Did Crystal have to be taken, too? My prayers ended with the plea, "God, don't let her die. Please don't let her die." Years later I was to understand why Crystal was allowed to enter eternity when she did and to thank God for his wisdom in taking her when he did.

One Sunday in January 1968, Crystal, Carol, and I were in our bedroom, making birthday cards for Mom. We were drawing birthday pictures on the floor with our crayons scattered round. Suddenly Crystal said, "I see two of you," and for minutes at a time, she began seeing double. Although I didn't know it at the time, her blood chemistry was going out of balance. But Mom and Dad knew and said that she would be going into the hospital in the morning.

We put our cards away and went downstairs to tell our parents that Crystal was seeing double. Crystal never finished that birthday card. Before the week was up she was dead.

That night, before she went into the hospital for the last time, as I was sitting in the living room in the evening, Crystal came and laid her head on my shoulder. I put my arm around her and leaned my head against hers. I remember thinking to myself, "What am I ever going to do if she dies?" and tears came into my eyes as I hugged her. Crystal turned and looked at me and said, "You're crying. Why?" I just shrugged it off as nothing. But I shall always cherish that moment when I think we both knew in our hearts what was coming but declined to express it. Yet more was said in those few moments without words than could ever be said with words.

On Monday morning Dad came upstairs and lifted Crystal out of bed. He and Mom took her to the hospital while Arthur, Carol, and I went to school.

Arthur and Carol took their lunch, because they were in high school, but Mom always made lunch for Dad and me as I came home at noon.

However, when one of the family was ill Mom sat by the bedside of the ill one day and night, sometimes enduring past exhaustion.

That week I came home and made lunch for Dad and myself, because Mom was at the hospital.

I'll never forget how heavy-hearted I was one day that week as I came home. I fixed beef noodle soup and sandwiches. As we were eating, I said to Dad, "I guess Crystal doesn't have very long to live." He replied, "What makes you think that?"

It turned out that at Dad's weekly Bible study some of the concerned parishioners had asked just exactly what Crystal's state of health was. Dad had told them that it looked as if Crystal had two weeks at the most. One of the parishioners had a daughter who was in my grade at school, although in another classroom. This parishioner had told her daughter the news. Her daughter had passed on the information at school. Consequently, one of my friends informed me.

Dad, when he heard this, was gentle with me and told me that it could be that she would rally and we might have her back with us for awhile longer. How I prayed that week! How I prayed for God to spare my little sister!

I didn't know at the time, but I found out later that when Mom and Dad brought Crystal in, Mom had alerted the top renal specialist at the University of Alberta Hospital. The specialist ordered bloodwork on Crystal's arrival and then assigned Crystal to his resident. The resident did not and could not know as much about advanced renal failure as the specialist. But the specialist doctor never even came to see Crystal once and showed no interest in her whatsoever. His nurse had told Mom that he would come; but then, when he saw Crystal's bloodwork results, he didn't bother.

Crystal came in on Monday and died on Friday. After she was dead, the head doctors showed interest in her—to do a biopsy. My parents refused.

Even being as young as I was, the specialist doctor is lucky I never met up with him because, if I had, there would have been one tremendous thunder and lightning session by one tiny thirteen-year-old girl!

I remember that on Friday night, Dad went to the hospital after supper. Mom was keeping her steady vigil there. He had told Carol that Crystal had gone into convulsions and the end was near. But to save me, I only knew that he would be going to see Crystal.

Yet I felt within me that things were not good. After they left, I turned on the television. The Smothers Brothers were on. Their humorous jokes seemed oppressive to me. I turned them off.

When Mom and Dad came home, I jumped for the door. "How's Crystal?" I asked. Mom quietly said, "Crystal has gone to heaven to be with Jesus." I just stared at her. Over and over again I cried out, "Not Crystal! No, not Crystal!"

Dad, Mom, Carol and I went into the living room as the tears began to fall. Arthur was next door babysitting; but as soon as he came home, he instantly knew what had happened. As we sat together, Dad raised Crystal's picture to the mantel where Eddie's and Grace's pictures were. "She's graduated to here now," he said. (The pictures of our loved ones that had passed on were on the mantel under the picture of Jesus that hung in the living room.)

Long after the others had stopped crying visibly, I sat in the corner of the chesterfield with my kleenex box, sobbing my heart out. It wasn't that I was grieving any more than the others; it was just that since Eddie and Grace had died when I was quite young, I hadn't yet learned to relinquish my sister's spirit into Jesus' hands until the day when we would all be reunited again.

The next few months were months that taught me about the pain of separation and the empty, achy feeling of grief and loneliness. Being young, these experiences were relatively new to me, and I felt them with great intensity.

Seeing the empty bed hurt, seeing the clothes hurt, and then always one would come upon some little reminder of Crystal which would bring on a new flood of tears.

At night I would dream that Crystal had come back. I would be so jubilant in my dreams and thank God that she wasn't dead after all. Then I would wake up to the reality. At times I dreamt that she came back and we were happy together. Then, suddenly she was gone. Once I dreamt that I was in the living room with her. She had on her furry-looking brown coat. She looked so cuddly in it that I went over and hugged her. That dream was a recreation of an actual experience.

In about March of that year, Mom and Dad could see that emotional stress was beginning to have an effect on my physical well-being.

I remember that Dad took me to school early in the morning one day for violin practice. As we were driving he told me that I mustn't grieve so much for Crystal. He went on to tell me of how heavily he had grieved for his first-born son—my brother Eddie. But one day, God gave him a dream that gave him new release.

Eddie came from heaven and met Dad on earth. Dad was overjoyed and they spent time talking together. But then Eddie said, "I have to go now, Dad. I have to go to choir practice." And so he returned to heaven.

Dad knew that Eddie was in glorious eternity with Jesus. He was experiencing what the Bible speaks about in I Corinthians 2:9, "What no eye has seen, nor ear heard, nor the heart of man conceived, what God has prepared for those who love Him."

But he realized after this dream that now Eddie would not want to come back even if he could because he had tasted of the glories of heaven and of life in eternity with his Savior, Jesus Christ. Dad told me that they couldn't come back to us; but one day, we could go to them. At this time, too, Mom gave me a tiny book entitled, A Little Book of Comfort.

One night, many months later, I was lying in bed, and from the depths of my heart I cried out, "Oh God, I miss that kid!" At that moment, I can honestly say that "heaven came down and glory filled my soul." A wonderful peace came into me and I felt that my heavy burden was being rolled away.

I began to think of Crystal, not as dead and gone, but very much alive and happy in heaven. She had taken the step that we all must take—that of leaving our physical bodies to enter into the spiritual realm of eternity. For her, it had come after less than eleven short years.

In March of that year, I began having pain in my ankle. I would be walking to school, and all of a sudden my ankle would get very painful to step on. Then it would swell up. I had to stay off my feet for the pain to leave.

Dad felt that maybe I had a sprained ankle and gave me some Absorbine Junior to rub on. But shortly after this, my other ankle began to swell in the same manner.

Our church was blocks from my home. On Saturday mornings my girl friend and I walked to church for Confirmation classes. I remember that halfway to the church, my ankle swelled up and it was painful to walk the rest of the way. It was hard to concentrate on the lesson that day because of the throbbing in my foot. After that, Dad drove me to class.

I also began to feel tired and listless. Mom realized that my kidneys were not functioning properly, and so she contacted our pediatrician. He, in turn, recommended me to the head renal specialist at the University of Alberta Hospital at the time.

My sister, Carol, had been under his care for some time. All through the years, from the time I was in grade three, Carol had been under doctors' care for renal failure and was in and out of the hospital. Throughout my childhood, there was fear many times that Carol would pass away. But in the end, Crystal was the one to go.

Once in the hospital, after many tests, I was put on the inevitable 40 gram protein diet since we were told that the kidneys could not handle heavy protein and the waste by-products associated with it. The amount of milk and meat consumption was reduced.

Because my kidneys were not functioning properly, they were excreting too much salt and so I was put on sodium bicarbonate pills and told to drink a lot of fluid to keep the kidneys flushed. This was my introduction to hospital life. It was the first of many, many sessions. During the summer, my ankles didn't swell up anymore, but a stiffness began to creep into my joints and my bones began to ache for periods at a time.

In the fall of 1969 I entered high school. I remember that in the first week of school the grade ten students would be rushing here and there to escape the frosh procedures of the grade twelve students. Exiting down a stairwell was a favorite escape. I joined the others, but I soon found that I couldn't run down the steps anymore and had to put a great deal of weight on the banister in order to go down the steps at any speed.

We went to a renal doctor to find out just what the trouble was. After having several x-rays my bone problem was diagnosed as renal rickets—the same bone pain that Crystal had suffered earlier. The doctor suggested massive doses of vitamin D in the hope that my kidneys would utilize some of the vitamins to restore calcium to my bones.

During this time, my brother Arthur was an active first year university student. He was a skilled pianist at an early age and had already taught piano at a certified music school. He was taking the Bachelor of Education degree program with a major in music.

It was in December of that year that the severe Hong Kong flu hit our city. Dad had it first and was very ill with it. Then Arthur got it. I remember he was in his bed all the time sleeping. Mom would bring him his meals, and when she saw that he was just eating mechanically she sensed that he was not totally conscious and feared that the flu had brought on severe kidney failure. Her fear was confirmed. Arthur's kidneys shut down, and he went into a coma. In order to save his life, he had to go on the artifical kidney machine. Tubes were put into his artery and vein surgically, and he went on the machine to have his blood cleansed in two twelve-hour sessions. And so began his life by means of an artificial support system.

By January of 1970, my bones had begun to deteriorate more rapidly. They ached continually and movement became painful. I remember that in a typing class, an elective I was taking, we had to type long exercises on manual typewriters. The electric typewriters came in a more advanced course. After several minutes of banging, my fingers hurt to pound the keys and my wrists began to ache. I started to have to put the weight of my body on my hands to get out of a chair. I also began to need blood transfusions because my bone marrow was not producing red cells in the way that it should.

The first time that I needed a blood transfusion, I was hospitalized for three days. Later, as they increased in frequency, I was sent to the dialysis unit. I remember that during my first trip to the unit for blood, I looked in a room with many beds in it. Dialysis treatment was very archaic at that time. Lying on the beds were very ill-looking people with yellow complexions. All around were transfusions, kidney basins, oxygen tanks, and saline bottles. I saw a man whose color was awful. His bones were so deformed. His chest stuck out like a barrel. Every bone seemed distorted. I could see the pain. I went into the side room to await the intravenous needle for my transfusion. I cried. I cried for him and for those people hooked to that machine who looked so ill, but who were trying so hard to live.

That summer, as the pain in my bones continued to increase because the calcium was leaving them, they became soft. My legs could no longer support my frame and I watched my ankles bend under the weight and slowly spread further and further apart. My knee joints also became bent.

By September my legs were bent quite badly. My feet were far apart when I stood with my knees together. Being in high school, I became very self-conscious and wore Carol's pants because they were much wider than my own. It took sheer determination and will-power to go to school that month. By the time I came home from school every evening, I was in tremendous pain and I could only manage baby steps.

My art class was on the first floor of the school. I left the class five minutes early in order to get to my literature class which was on the next floor. It was painful to get to a standing position. Every step hurt and I slowly took the stairs one at a time.

Even with starting out early, the door was closed to my next class before I got there. I remember opening the door while the whole class watched. I slowly made my way to my chair. I heard a boy say, "Look at the way she walks!" and laugh.

Towards the end of the day, every step was effort. The halls would be swarming at class break. I'll never forget how some boys behind me swore because with the swell of students they couldn't pass me and had to be content to go at a snail's pace.

When I came home I had a bath in very hot water which helped to ease the pain. But at night my bones felt as if little insects were burrowing into them. At the end of September I told Mom that I couldn't live with the pain any longer; and if something weren't done, my life would soon be over.

All during this time, I went consistently to the hospital to have bloodwork taken as my blood chemistry—especially my sodium and potassium levels were regulated through the use of huge salt pills, sodium bicarbonate, and occasionally potassium liquid. Eight to ten tubes of blood were taken for the purpose of blood chemistry regulation. But I found out years later from a resident that many tubes were saved over the years to study the progress of my disease. The loss of blood caused my hemoglobin to fall and increased the frequency of blood transfusions.

Mom contacted the doctor and asked if anything could be done for my fast-deteriorating condition. My x-rays showed that my bones had gotten very thin and fragile. He told her that a certain doctor had come up with a new theory. Since the kidneys were not functioning properly, the parathyroid glands had taken over and were secreting a hormone which was forcing the calcium to leave the bones, thus causing rickets. He felt that if the parathyroid glands were removed and calcium was administered intravenously, the bones would then be able to accept the calcium if there was enough kidney function for vitamin D to be metabolized by the kidney. This was because the kidney metabolizes vitamin D into another form. This metabolized form causes the bones to accept the calcium.

This total parathyroidectomy, as it was called, had never been done on a kidney patient in the University Hospital. Then there was the question of whether or not my kidneys were strong enough to take anesthetic and the surgery without shutting down.

Mom asked the doctor, "Would you let your daughter have this surgery?" He replied in the affirmative. When Mom approached me about the surgery, I said that it had to be done. I couldn't carry on as I was.

I was hospitalized in the children's ward in October. I was fifteen.

I was taken for an intravenous pyelogram—a test where a colored fluid was injected and then scans of the kidney were taken by x-ray. This test revealed that I had milliary cystic kidneys. There were hundreds of little cysts in my kidneys.

The doctor took me down to a doctor's meeting where the pros and cons of my surgery were discussed, since this surgery would be a first in the hospital. Together we slowly made our way down the elevator and inched toward the doctors' room. I sat outside while I was being discussed.

I was called in and after answering questions I was asked to walk up the aisle to demonstrate just how bent my legs had become. Then I was allowed to leave. It was decided that I should go through with the surgery.

Somehow, as I sat in my hospital bed I felt that I wasn't going to live through this surgery. I really struggled with this. I read my Bible and prayed, and told God that I felt I was going to die, but that I didn't want to die yet. In the quiet hours of the evening, I struggled and wrestled with this in prayer.

Soon afterward I had a dream which made me feel that I wasn't going to die. There was a peaceful tranquil mauve sort of haze in my dream. I saw Jesus on the cross and behind Him there was a boy and two girls. I knew that they were Eddie, Grace, and Crystal.

When I woke up I remembered the dream. I felt it meant that since I wasn't there, my time had not come. However, I came very, very close to death shortly after the surgery.

The attending surgeon came to discuss the surgery with me. He told me that a slit would be made at the base of my neck and the four glands would be removed. He asked me if there were any questions. I asked if I could keep the glands. The answer was no.

I still remember waking up in the recovery room. A nurse asked how I felt. I squeaked out in a hoarse whisper, "My throat hurts."

For ten consecutive days and nights I was given bottle after bottle of intravenous calcium. My bones soaked it up.

It had turned out that in the operating room, three of my parathyroid glands were found. But the fourth one could not be found. Finally part of my thymus gland was also removed and the fourth parathyroid gland was found embedded in it. All of my glands were very enlarged.

The danger after the surgery was that of tetany—if the serum calcium in the blood dropped too low, with no glands, there was no bodily regulatory system to elevate the calcium if it went too low. After this ten day period my blood was constantly checked, because I would get tingling in my fingers, a sign of tetany or convulsions when the calcium drops too low.

When I was up and around again, I phoned Mom and told her that I would be having a bath. She worried about this because she felt that if I were alone and in water, and my calcium dropped, there could be serious consequences. She phoned the doctor, and he said there was nothing to worry about.

After my bath I felt strange. I went to the desk and told the nurse; but I couldn't lay a finger on just what was wrong. She told me to lie down on my bed for awhile. Although the next 17½ hours of my life will always remain blank, I went into convulsions right at the main desk, and the battle for my life began. This was at 10:00 in the morning. I remember waking up once and seeing my renal specialist with several doctors and nurses all around. I asked him to phone my mother.

He didn't phone her until 1:00 and then he said that she had better come. I remained unconscious, and in the evening, Arthur, Carol, and Dad came up. There was uncertainty as to whether or not I would be alive in the morning.

The patient beside me, a younger girl whom I had come to know, was moved out and Mom was given the bed to sleep on so that she could be near me through the night. A special nurse was assigned to me for the night shift.

At 3:30 in the morning, I awoke and tried to speak, but my tongue wouldn't cooperate and all that came out was garbled mumbo jumbo.

The night nurse who kept vigil hugged Mom for joy. She was so glad that I had made it. By the morning I was again speaking but every muscle in my body felt as if it had been stretched out of shape. I was hooked to intravenous calcium after that, and when it was disconnected a syringe and calcium were kept close at hand so that a shot of calcium could be injected into my bloodstream if my serum calcium dropped too low once again.

Not long after, I was talking to the patient in the bed next to me when my tongue got thick again. But an intravenous injection cleared it up before anything serious had developed.

I got talking to a resident one day. He told me that since my bones were accepting calcium, they would begin to harden. However, since they were bent, they would harden in a bent form, and then it would be too late to straighten my limbs. He felt that I should get braces or casts put on my legs so that they would heal in a straight position. I thought a lot about this. It made sense to me.

Shortly after, I made my way down the corridor to the doctor's office. He happened to be in. I remember sitting down in the chair offered to me. The doctor said, "It must be pretty important to come all this way," since he knew of the pain that I had to walk. I explained my problem and asked for casts to be put on my legs.

The doctor told me that there were drawbacks. It took months for the calcium to leave my bones and for my bones to become soft and bend. He said that if casts were put on first of all, the bones would have to be reset and then that they would only bend again if taken out of the cast. However, there was a glimmer of hope. Although I was fifteen, my body, because of the kidney disease, had not developed as fast as it should have developed. My bones were, therefore, still growing. If the calcium went back into my bones and my bones began to harden, my bones, on their own, would heal and begin to straighten.

We looked at my legs. The knees were quite enlarged and from there to my ankles looked like an upside down V with my feet turned outwards at the ends. I remember saying, "It will just take time then?" He nodded and said, "Time and patience."

That year I missed a lot of school. The calcium levels in my bloodstream would suddenly drop, and sometimes in the middle of the night I had to go to the emergency ward for intravenous calcium. In the winter months Dad would warm up the car and take Mom and me to the hospital.

Although my legs didn't straighten quickly, they accepted calcium very fast. When you lose something like your mobility, you don't take walking for granted very easily again. It was such a relief to open a car door without pain, or to roll down a car window or—blessed relief—to lie down without aching.

My x-rays showed continued acceptance of calcium and strengthening of my bones. I could finally climb stairs without pain and walk normally again. I continued to have hospital sessions in grade twelve to regulate the chemical balance in my blood; but with mobility restored, they were easier to endure.

In late December or early January of grade twelve, I developed a severe headache. The doctor said to bring me to the hospital but could find nothing severely out of balance. However, he said that I should stay in the hospital for a few days for observation. That few days lasted one month. During this time a resident doctor was allowed to look after me. He took many blood tests but not much more.

I was taking salt tablets at the time because my kidneys could not retain salt. With the salt tablets I was on, the sodium level in my bloodstream was maintained.

The resident decided to take me off the salt pills. Since an order was an order at the hospital, my salt tablets were discontinued accordingly. Of course, my muscles cramped and I began to get very dizzy, to be sick to my stomach, and to get very weak because the sodium level in my blood dropped to dangerously low levels. The salt pills were restored.

At that time, I began to get pain in my ankles so x-rays were taken. I still remember the doctor coming to my room and asking me if I had ever thought about dialysis.

I replied that it had crossed my mind but that was years away. The doctor told me that the x-rays were showing signs of bone deterioration again, and it looked as if the artificial kidney machine would be a reality sooner than I thought.

After he left, I remember lying with my head at the foot of the bed and my feet resting at the top of the headboard. I thought for a time and then I said to my roommate who had multiple sclerosis, "If I get bone disease again. . .I think I'll give up."

She said, "No, you won't. You'll carry on." In all sincerity I said, "No, I really don't think so." How glad I am that in January of grade twelve, I could not see into the future.

When I wrote my first departmental exams, the blood urea poisoning was very high. Normal BUN in the blood is 8–20; mine was 160. I would forget things easily. I was needing more and more salt pills but because of all the salt, my blood pressure started to rise to the point where tiny vessels would burst. Consequently, I would get severe nose bleeds and blood transfusions were becoming more frequent. Once I convulsed at home.

In February, I was readmitted. I no longer felt like eating, and I was becoming more and more ill. My sister Carol was also in hospital and was preparing to go on dialysis because her kidney function was also stopping.

I remember that the doctor came to my room and told me that the time had come for me to go on hemodialysis. He said that first of all I would have a 48-hour-treatment of peritoneal dialysis. A tube would be inserted into my stomach and fluid circulated through. This fluid, after a period, would then be drained and the process would be repeated. Finally, I would be taken to surgery for a cannula and then, hemodialysis would begin.

~   ~   ~   ~

CHAPTER 2

HEARTBEAT WRAPPED WITH PLASTIC

Did I but live nearer to God,
I could be of so much more help.

—George Hodges

Past Lives

During more than forty years, kidney disease has been a way of life for our family. Two brothers and three sisters are no longer alive. I continue to live because of the artificial kidney machine, a machine which cleanses my blood of impurities that build up due to non-functioning kidneys. I want to share with you our experiences of illness—the experiences on the artificial kidney machine that have dramatically changed the quality of our lives, written during our pioneering years on dialysis, 1969 to 1975.

When I was ten years old, Mother told me that I had kidney failure. I understood this in terms of Edward's life, my oldest brother who had died two years earlier. Kidney failure meant trips to the hospital, bad tasting medicine, riding in a wheelchair and eating as much fresh fruit as I wanted. Mother's sorrow spilled over to me—I climbed upstairs, lay on my bed and wept. Finally I stood up and resolved, "I will never cry about this again."

In the years that followed, kidney failure became a private world: I never shared my experiences with school friends. However, I spent time in the hospital, there was bad tasting medicine to take, and sometimes I rode in a wheelchair because I was too weak to walk. But a low protein diet was in vogue instead of the fresh fruit diet. By the time I was in high school, it became apparent that I was not the only one in our family with kidney failure. How can I express our family's anxiety as we watched Joy's bones deteriorate; our aching sorrow when Crystal died; our distress when the Hong Kong flu caused Arthur to begin treatments on the artificial kidney machine? I wondered about our future.

Machine Life

Shortly after Arthur began hemodialysis treatments, I had my first blood transfusion, another signal of my worsening condition. I was at the Artificial Kidney Unit for the transfusion. In the hall, I met one of the people whose life was maintained by the artificial kidney machine. He was hunch-backed and barrel-chested with advanced bone deterioration because of kidney failure. He was thin and anemic. His eyes were glazed with the knowledge of suffering. He smiled at me.

In the nine-bed ward, blood for transfusions was hanging from a couple of poles, someone was throwing up, the smell of formaldehyde and body odor permeated the place. Most of the people were paler than death—lips blanched of any color, with sallow complexions. Yet, they laughed easily and enjoyed each other's company. They held jobs. It seemed to me they were living in spite of the machine. And Arthur was one of them. He continued his studies at the university. At home, after his twelve-hour hemodialysis treatments, he literally crawled up the stairs in the entry; then collapsed on the sofa, gasping for air. Joy and I watched him, fearful he would die any minute. I told Joy, "I'd rather die than go on the artificial kidney machine." I meant it.

In his first year of university, Arthur found himself coming out of a three day semi-conscious lapse. The function of his kidneys was minimal, and by February of 1969 he was faced with continuing life only by resorting to an artificial life-support system, the artificial kidney machine. To submit himself to total dependence on the machine was very difficult;

however, his only alternative was death, and the desire for life made such a submission possible.

While on his first treatment, Arthur was introduced to two patients. To the left lay a young man with a deformed body and bags connected to collect his urine. On the other side was a young man who refused to greet him and turned his face to the wall. He suffered depression and ignored both staff and patients. To see what his future might include in terms of both physical and psychological well-being was horrifying. Arthur prayed and committed himself to the hands of God, trusting that he would guide and keep him through his uncertain future on the kidney machine. God's peace flooded Arthur's soul.

Energy was completely lacking because his hemoglobin, like that of many companions on the machine, was very low. Arthur required more and more transfused blood in order to survive. To move about gasping for air and having to sit down after moving short distances or walking up or down a few stairs, can only be described as survival. Sitting on steps, garbage cans, and heat registers in order to gain the needed oxygen for equilibrium on his way to classes at the university was routine. Arthur overheard the description, "Walking dead man," more than once. But he wasn't alone. Our father took the time from his busy schedule to assist him into an obsolete freight elevator countless times at the Arts Building of the University in order to spare him the fifty-two stairs—when stairs become mountains, you count them.

One day on his way to university classes, after dialyzing all night, Arthur heard a kidney unit doctor speaking over the car radio. He stated that people on the kidney machine lived a "near normal life." Yes, but accomplishments were in spite of the machine, resulting from sheer determination rather than energy.

In the fall of 1969, Arthur's eyes became infected which later resulted in a hemorrhage in one eye because of a doctor's wrong diagnosis and high blood pressure. He became blind in that eye and the infection left him with twenty percent vision in the other. Arthur counted heavily upon his hearing in his second year of university and was granted oral assignments and exams. Here again, our family provided the necessary help at a time when it was desperately needed. For example, my mother read textbooks to Arthur in the evenings. The trauma and concern of those days were great.

In the spring of 1970, Arthur became ill with a liver infection. It became crystal clear to the family that his physical deterioration was only worsening ever since he had begun hemodialysis. He was not alone. Many patients, particularly those who lived by means of regular interval blood transfusions, faced the same reality. Many resorted to kidney transplants believing them to be their only alternative. Indeed, what other alternatives did we have?

Transplantation has been an integral part of treatment of chronic renal failure patients at our kidney unit. In the summer of 1969, a transplant immunology laboratory was established with one and a quarter million to spend in a period of five years. More grants have continued coming to keep this program going.

The primary difficulty of kidney transplantation was spelled out in 1958 by a kidney specialist at the Mayo Clinic in Rochester, Minnesota to my father who was trying to secure help for Edward, my oldest brother, who was close to death. The doctor explained that the body fights to reject an organ foreign to itself. He likened the process of kidney transplant rejection to a sliver in a finger which the body attempts to discharge. The doctor could not be optimistic. He stated that medical science might never solve the problems of rejection; however, the possibility was here.

Many years later the problem of rejection as it relates to kidney transplants still exists. Although the longest functioning transplant from our kidney unit in 1973 was over five years, many patients have taken the risky step and lost. The working transplant is not without its problems either. The heavy medications necessary to keep the body from rejecting the transplanted kidney take their toll in various side effects and problems, some of which cause immeasurable suffering and death. But there are those who have been fortunate enough to enjoy some relatively good years of life on transplants.

In March of 1970, our family resolved to use common sense in all facets of our treatment and therefore initiate a degree of individual care. In so doing we were in fuller control of our lives on the machine. We had always attempted to learn everything about kidney disease and its treatment. Arthur was the first in our family on the machine. I was to be second.

My life during my second year of university was increasingly incongruous with the reality that I was dying a little each day. Blood samples were taken weekly so that the blood chemistry could be balanced by medication; later, I discovered that many extra tubes were taken for use in research even though my hemoglobin was maintained at a gradually lower level by transfused blood. The impurities in the blood continued to rise and there was nothing to be done. I began to compare my existence with the life-style on the machine. I knew that my blood chemistry could be balanced and maintained with hemodialysis. Also, the nausea and fatigue that Arthur suffered were increasingly a part of my daily existence. Yet, I would not yield my life to the machine. I dreaded being a part of the sallow-faced group who existed in the no-man's land between life and death. In February 1971, I finally put my life in God's hands and ceased trying to work out my own destiny. I accepted the artificial kidney machine as the means of my existence. In the same week that I began hemodialysis, my sister Joy was told that she, too, must begin.

My Mother's Response to Illness

Arthur had been on dialysis since February 1969. Two years later, also in February, Carol and Joy were both admitted to the hospital in preparation for the beginning of dialysis.

Carol and Joy had been more fortunate than the great majority of kidney patients in delaying the beginning of dialysis. We had inevitably endured a long conflict in an effort to have full access to results from our blood tests. Once that right was irretrievably established (after having had the privilege periodically withdrawn), we could proceed to establish a sensible pattern of diet according to individual differences. And very marked differences they were, even for siblings. How many months or years earlier they would otherwise have had to depend on a machine for dialysis, we do not know.

Once in the hospital, we were suddenly victims of a research bureaucracy which, we sensed, was by no means benevolent. That bloodthirsty research monster demanded its endless take, and time and time again the blood technician came to carry out her orders to extract blood. No amount of remonstration deterred doctor, nurse or laboratory technician. Of course, we recognize the fact that nurses and technicians are subordinate to doctors and simply follow orders.

There was the day that Carol was taken into a sideroom to have blood taken for various tests. About ten tubes were drawn—about one hundred cubic centimeters according to Carol's estimate—with the result that she was so weakened that she could not rise. After this experience came the days of struggling with added weakness and dizziness and the almost futile attempt to build enough blood to function.

This particular episode occurred before Carol was on dialysis and during the period before she had blood transfusions. Her hemoglobin at that time was a little better than one-half normal.

This added affliction of the loss of much blood that she, as a kidney patient could not readily replace was, obviously, not to Carol's advantage. Numerous statistics were undoubtedly gathered, but this particular episode hastened her collapse.

All kidney patients in the 1971 period experienced the hardship of low hemoglobin. Joy and Carol were then dependent on transfusions for survival. This was also true of Arthur. To me it was sadly obvious that Carol and Joy were being depleted of blood and strength to the extent that their encounter with the dialysis machine would be most hazardous and difficult. Without the excessive blood loss, the ordeal would have been more than rigorous at best.

My heart sank like lead when I entered Joy's ward one day. She said that she had reached a condition of weakness and fatigue of such magnitude that she could not raise her head. So utterly sapped of strength was she that we silently despaired of the immediate future. How could her emaciated little body possibly survive the rigors of the first dialysis ordeal?

The day—yes, numerous successive dialysis days—came when Joy paid the price. Again and again came those agonizing days with an extra suffering penalty needlessly attached. If only we could relive them after having acquired the knowledge that is now ours. How very, very much unnecessary misery could have been avoided.

Darkness Threatens

Distressing news of various kinds had become quite frequent at our house and, admittedly, adjustments had to be made. Sometimes these adjustments came by no means readily. This particular day was to be no exception.

It was in 1970 in the beginning of Arthur's second year at the university and his second year on dialysis. I had just returned from a women's meeting. Arthur informed me that he had seen a trickle of blood running down the back of his eyes. He had informed his doctor when this happened during the dialysis. The doctor, a nephrologist, insisted that Arthur could not possibly see blood on the back of his eye and concluded that it must be mucus. Arthur was very unhappy about the whole incident, but had found his persuasive powers insufficient to convince the doctor that his vision was at stake.

Arthur was not the only unhappy one by this time. I went to the telephone to call the doctor. Fortunately, the nephrologist was in his office. Our concern was obviously not distressing him to the same degree. He conceded that an appointment had been made by his secretary for Arthur to see the ophthalmologist the following Thursday! There was no inkling of immediate concern or urgency. The following Thursday was six days away.

Immediately, I telephoned the chief ophthalmologist at our hospital and stated our concerns. He replied that he was having his office location changed, and that he was in the midst of moving. He, therefore, seemed very reluctant to bestir himself. "Now or never," I said. There was no choice in such an emergency situation.

In a matter of minutes Arthur and his father were in the ophthalmologist's office. Soon they returned home with the sombre verdict. The eye doctor had fully elaborated on Arthur's deteriorated condition. He couldn't produce his own blood; furthermore, his bones were deteriorating. And now, according to this eye doctor, his vision would definitely be lost. True, his eyes were sorely afflicted with infection. His sober prognosis was that Arthur's life was nearing its end and that blindness would be inevitable. There was only one hope in the form of an experimental venture. Cortisone injections in both eyes were to be tried as a new procedure, but he surmised that procedure might serve the purpose.

This solution sounded preposterous to us. We went into family conference as we always had done when major decisions had to be made. We would under no circumstances accept blindness as inevitable.

Our reasoning proceeded thus. If we permitted both eyes to be injected with cortisone, Arthur may then certainly be blinded in both eyes. If neither eye was injected and he became blind as predicted, we would blame ourselves for ignoring the medical professional remedy offered. The decision was unanimous. We would permit the ophthalmologist to inject only one eye with cortisone.

To this day we regret that decision. Were we in the same situation again without the knowledge we have, there would seem to be no rational alternative. After all, the eye doctor had been very adamant. Surely he could, at least, have consulted other senior eye doctors in such a grave predicament. Any patient would be in a state of quandary under similar pressuring circumstances. Hindsight is always a little clearer than foresight.

The ophthalmologist had thought it incredible that the nephrologist had diagnosed the bleeding in the eye as mucus. We thought it incredible that the ophthalmologist would offer such extreme treatment as an experimental cortisone injection in the eyeball.

The eye pierced with the needle of cortisone hemorrhaged during a subsequent dialysis session. Arthur wished to discontinue dialysis short of full time to safeguard his eye to that extent at least, since the heparin setting was apparently too high.

Naturally, blood-thinner, such as heparin, must always be used to prevent the artificial kidney from clotting, but it was logical that eye blurring and threat of hemorrhage should have dictated discontinuance of dialysis treatment on that particular day. It was another error for which Arthur was to pay the cost in lack of normal vision for a long, long time to come. The eye that had been injected with cortisone became progressively weaker in vision whereas the other eye became slowly but gradually stronger.

And how does one continue one's studies at the university without sufficient sight to see the blackboard, to read the textbooks, and to write? Where there is a will, there is usually a way, even though it may by no means be an easy one. Where there is hope, there is courage to press on.

So it was that I became Arthur's home tutor and secretary. During classes at the university he could not see what the professor wrote on the blackboard. At home, he could not read his textbooks. Neither could he write. He was at the mercy of circumstances and those in his rather limited sphere of activity.

To professors at the University of Alberta we owe a debt of gratitude. So much consideration was given by many of them. Arthur had to submit to oral examinations which are considerably more difficult than written examinations. It was a taxing ordeal for busy professors, too, with scores of students and as many examination papers to mark. Eventually, the time came when he was able to write part of the examination and complete the remainder orally. Subject after subject was thus completed and his credits accrued.

During this period Arthur acquired an exceptionally good memory. I recall telling him that it was impossible to read the book material aloud to him more than once because there

was so much to be read and so little time to accomplish what
had to be done. The dialysis treatments then were very trying
and demanded also much time. Twelve hours were spent on
dialysis in addition to preparation for dialysis and work on
the machine afterwards. Much of the time he was too ill to
do anything because of this faulty treatment in over-dialysis.
It seemed that we had to accomplish twice as much in
proportion to the time normally allotted to students.

To give up was unthinkable. Each success that we
experienced together spurred us on to greater and more
scheduled endeavor. Our time-table continued to be very
flexible and very full. It must constantly be borne in mind
that a kidney patient has much less time as a student to
accomplish his studies. During the gruelling dialysis sessions
of those days before the reforms that we struggled so long
to obtain, the aftermath of dialysis was exhaustion in the
extreme. In the few hours of normal living after recovery from
dialysis until the next dialysis, so much had to be accomplished. The demands of the kidney machine had to come first
in those dreadful days, and the chores of life had to be
sandwiched in between. That we managed so surprisingly
well in spite of such heavy odds is largely attributable to a
doggedness of determination and purpose that would not give
in no matter how great the cost.

There is nothing that so drives a drained body as a
determined mind. But behind the limited physical and mental
resources were the spiritual resources of a supernatural
supply. Prayer to our Creator reminded us that He was also
our preserver.

Arthur was majoring in music at the university. Because
of his eyesight deficiency, the notes had to be drawn the size
of marbles with a felt pen. As time went on, vision was
gradually and partially restored in the one eye that had not
been pierced by a cortisone needle.

I will always remember the seemingly endless reading
of music history that was a source of delight to Arthur. A most
fascinating course on Russia in political science required
countless hours of reading. When my throat needed rest, a

cup of coffee would usually suffice for restoration of my voice. Then we would again proceed.

And so the hours and days and months passed. Much was achieved in those days when darkness threatened. Pressing on toward a goal with a meaningful purpose assuaged the pain of many a heartache. Gainful occupation of the mind left little time for self-contemplation, and that was a blessing indeed.

Every now and then Arthur was required to make return visits to the eye doctor. The eye would be frozen somehow so it did not move, then examined under strong light. It was a trying ordeal. The medical students would be called in for observation. Such an eye was really different! Finally it dawned on us that a halt must be called to this stressful and excessive examination. There was no cure available. There was no way in which Arthur stood to gain or benefit by these frequent performances. No good for us had ever come out of that office. We left it never to return. Instead we secured the services of a most careful and capable optometrist for whose dedication we were so grateful.

This optometrist friend, so kind and concerned, marvelled that Arthur could see well enough to teach music all day long. This doctor has done excellently in the fitting of lenses that helped so much in light control. The greatest asset was that Arthur was no longer primarily a research object.

Research Objects

Kidney patients were relegated to the category of research objects in no uncertain terms. Blood was used freely for testing, and heavy demands were otherwise made upon a patient's time and energy for many frequently repeated testing endeavors other than those that were blood-related. Added to all the time-consuming testing was the incessant pressure to submit to various procedures, much unnecessary surgery, and the frequent demands to use various hormones.

Blood Tests

Before me, as I write, is a charting sheet indicating the monthly testing to be done for blood as well as routine tests used by our public kidney unit. Listed are sodium, potassium, chloride, calcium, phosphorous, magnesium, blood urea nitrogen, creatinine, uric acid, alkaline phosphatase, SGOT, LDH, bilirubin, Australian antigen, iron, total iron binding capacity, cytotoxicity, and hemoglobin. Others not listed on the sheet but sometimes taken were, WBC, carbon dioxide, total protein, albumin, glucose, and serum cholesterol.

The monthly blood testing was usually done before and after the last monthly dialysis. It was dreaded because of the blood-loss causing weakness and the feeling of a generally rundown condition. The knowledge that blood-building ability was at a dangerous low did not improve the morale.

Common sense dictated that an attempt be made to halt Arthur's rapid physical deterioration in the autumn of his year in grade ten. This was clearly the responsibility with priority at that particular time.

Aware that a knowledge of the bloodwork would help us in determining the best type of care as far as food and medication were concerned, the youngsters were periodically checked by our pediatrician. He, in turn, advised us to go to the kidney specialist who simply repeated the blood tests already done. This double loss of blood in liberal quantity was considerable indeed for anemic children. Naturally we were distressed.

One day the realization that this waste of blood must be prevented drove us to action. The urologist was then informed that the blood tests would be done once and not repeated. He disagreed. He felt we should proceed as before with the 'double take.' The consequences would be ours to bear; therefore, we made the decision. From then on, blood was taken only once for tests.

The experiences through the months and years ahead made it abundantly clear that our decision was right. The patient has a right to benefit from the preservation of blood so vital to life and physical welfare. Low hemoglobins would only be further decreased by blood loss causing greater weakness.

The blood is the river of life. Its condition must inevitably be determined because the results of tests are a revelation of the condition of the body. Therefore our motto became, "minimum testing for maximum benefits."

In desperation we then requested our urologist to consider what course to follow to determine progress of the disease. Recession or a halt—even a temporary one—were, hopefully, possibilities.

The urologist put Arthur in hospital and ordered morning blood tests in generous quantity. Arthur was well enough to move about as freely as he pleased, and made use of his freedom to explore the wards and make friends. At high school, classes went on as usual without him, and he was inevitably getting behind in his work.

This time our doctor was requested to release Arthur from the hospital in order to resume his studies. He readily agreed but stipulated that Arthur must be brought daily to the hospital before the day's classes in order to continue the blood tests.

This procedure, too, went on and on. Even though it seemed difficult to probe for truth as to what was happening, it was determined that any failure to ascertain that truth would not be due to any lack of effort on our part. Thereupon, I telephoned the blood laboratory and inquired as to what was being done with Arthur's blood. Instead of demanding a check with our doctor according to our expectation, a cheerful voice proceeded to narrate an interesting episode.

Arthur's blood, the voice explained, was being collected in quantity to be shipped to Montreal. "A large batch" was the term used. But, explained the voice, the whole "batch had spoiled; therefore, a new batch" was being collected and, when a sufficient quantity would have been again collected, that new batch would be shipped to Montreal.

In disbelief I clung to the receiver. In spite of my state of shock, sufficient presence of mind remained to advise the laboratory technician that his service would no longer be needed for this particular project. He, of course, was simply obeying the order of a senior.

The situation was duly pondered and assessed. Arthur, as you have already surmised, had suffered the double loss of blood and school time. It became our urgent duty to endeavor to restore him to his former condition, such as it was, before we sought the help of our doctor. We, as parents, and Arthur, as a student and patient, had wasted much time and effort, and the results were lamentable as far as Arthur was concerned. Unwittingly, he had been used for research to his own chagrin. It was not to be his last experience of such a nature.

Practices of this kind, in what we term 'blood extortion' to the detriment of the patient, were factors with which we were long to contend. At the time of this writing, the struggle for our rights has been won in regard to blood testing, but there were many skirmishes before that achievement.

X-rays

On the charting sheet were also listed the following routine tests: nerve conduction, when ordered; skeletal survey, every six months; chest x-ray, every six months; ECG (electrocardiogram), every six months; technetium scan, when ordered; and echocardiogram, when ordered.

The frequency with which skeletal survey requisitions arrived was startling. Each survey consisted of sixteen exposures and as many retakes as necessary. The degree of risk for kidney patients from radiation, however low-level it might be, was not known but feared by thinking patients. Certainly deteriorating bones were also subjected to added risk.

Our children, particularly Joy, when still little more than a child, would welcome the skeletal survey as something that was painless. She frequently angered the doctors by refusing avoidable painful procedures that would not benefit her but would give the doctors more statistics. She looked upon yielding to skeletal surveys as a peace-making device that would serve to appease any lingering wrath over numerous refusals. Statistics were to be compiled regardless of the patient's welfare. One doctor used to comment, "It's good for the statistics."

The time came when we decided as a family to remain adamant in our determination to bring skeletal surveys to a halt. The arguments against our decision were many, and insistence to resume such x-ray checking was constant. Finally, I telephoned the x-ray department to request a complete listing of all skeletal surveys and all other x-rays together with dates for each family member on dialysis. That request could not be granted by anyone in the x-ray department without a doctor's order.

But no doctor was willing to comply with the request. That x-ray statement for our family would have been a revelation indeed, but to this day it has not arrived.

Surgeries

Then, there were the surgeries, some of which were necessary, and most of which were unnecessary. Some hemodialysis people had altogether too many and too frequent operation room ordeals.

I well recall the chief transplant doctor going from bed to bed, checking the spleens of our three young people. The frequent blood transfusions seemed to cause the spleen to swell, and that could be easily felt by an experienced hand. Splenectomies were purported to cause rise in hemoglobin.

Whenever hesitancy was expressed by our young people in regard to surgery or other procedures, the answer was that success had been so very evident in Montreal or in some other distant place. In time we came to the conclusion that the rosy reports applicable elsewhere were not to be matched by our kidney unit. Distant pastures often appear to be greener.

Our young people soon decided that splenectomies were not for them. Nor were the bilateral nephrectomies so much warned against in some medical journal articles. Nor were the bone biopsies, two of which were needed as a minimum for comparison. They feared the fate of bone patients who became immobilized after their bone biopsies. The kidney biopsies too were avoided. Carol had one in the early years (about 1962) nine years before she began dialysis, and nothing definite was determined by that ordeal. The saphenous vein graft, an access for dialysis, was a procedure for which two of our young people endured pressure, but the folly of that route was all too obvious; that procedure has long been obsolete.

Then there was the bovine graft that so often burst, sending blood to the ceiling. The common fistula, too, we avoided because the insertion of two large needles three times weekly was in itself a traumatic experience. The persistent bleeding after the removal of the two needles was a plague too; many infections often resulted. The cannula was our life-line. Though painless on dialysis, there was the ever-present danger of the arterial or venous connection loosening, even though securely sutured and embedded in the flesh. As for parathyroidectomies, our family pioneered them. They were to serve insofar as possible until Dr. De Luca's bone drug would eventually relieve the wretchedness of bone pain and deformity.

Common Sense Research

By September 1971, Arthur had suffered the wretched-ness of dialysis, as it was then, for over two and one-half years. Joy and Carol were in their seventh month.

Something had to be done since the frequent visits to the doctors' offices in person or by telephone achieved so very little. A number of issues were thus kept more or less con-tinuously in the limelight, and that in itself was significant. It occurred to us that we could accomplish nothing unless we could penetrate the armor of the man who had the overall responsibility. He also had the power. An appointment was made.

The task was no less than colossal. We decided to initially settle for three major changes as a very substantial beginning. From there, the reform program could conceivably progress. Our three requests, together with our rationalizations, would be a hematocrit machine, fewer hours on the machine, and distilled water.

The day of the appointment inevitably came. I proceeded down steps inside the hospital that led me underground and eventually through a passage into a large room where I noticed a blackboard. Familiar names of kidney patients were listed on it in regard to what medical procedure was under consideration. I noted our son's name in particular and had my suspicions verified as to what his future should be. Beyond that room I was ushered into a wee office—by no means an ostentatious room for the world-renowned doctor I was soon to encounter.

Finally, he appeared. I waited for the ordeal to begin. It was soon apparent that he was not inclined to yield on any issue. Timewise, he was unusually generous. Clocks seem to be without hands in a hospital setting, but not usually in doctor's offices.

I was up to bat. I had three strikes and a fabulous, not-to-be-contested OUT! after each strike. Then the doctor with the overall responsibility for transplantation informed me that he had discussed our family's needs with his two chief nephrologists. I had supposed the appointment to be personal and confidential. Not so! He had chosen to have a meeting with his men before meeting with me. Their unanimous decision had been to offer a transplant. My answer was a predetermined No.

The world-renowned doctor irately replied that Arthur would be of age in a very short time (actually the following month), and then he could make his own decision. And, I may add, he did not fail to keep his word, but his undaunted efforts were to be of no avail.

I went home after the interview utterly defeated but more determined than ever to bring about reforms so obviously needful. Yes, the contest for what we knew to be right would go relentlessly on. The three initial goals—a hematocrit machine, fewer hours, and distilled water—were to be achieved in full measure, but the waiting period for each was to be long and difficult.

Pure Water

Because hours on dialysis were so needlessly many when Arthur began dialysis treatment in February 1969, and the equipment was poorly maintenanced as well, we felt that quality of life could and surely would improve. But how? There must be a better way. We must find it, and that must be soon. The death toll at the public kidney unit was heavy, and suffering was everywhere present.

Every now and then we talked as a family about the possibilities of clean distilled water when we were at home, as well as to doctors, whenever the situation presented itself to pursue the topic. Nothing ever came of it.

Oftentimes, we would continue to ponder the advisability of using tap water in our machines. The Edmonton Journal sometimes made reference to the fact that city water was by no means as desirable as it might be. Therefore, in September 1971, the appointment was made with the transplant doctor to introduce and, hopefully, try distilled water.

This particular doctor had replied that distilled water had been tried in Winnipeg, but no improvement had been indicated. He felt that the use of distilled water was not something to be pursued. Certainly he saw no reason for trying such a venture in Edmonton. He displayed no interest whatsoever.

Transplant surgery was this doctor's solution. Arthur was an expensive patient to maintain. The burden of cost to the hospital was a point of frequent and painful reference. Arthur could not produce his own blood, bone deterioration was serious, and his vision was minimal. But Arthur could be converted from a hospital liability to a research asset by accepting a twenty thousand dollar transplant. Secretly, I wondered if transplantation was not only this transplant doctor's primary concern but his only concern as well. I began to sense a steeled and cold hardness in this researcher. Perhaps, he was totally calloused to the needs of dialysis patients. He had, after all, suggested that the number of dialysis hours be increased to fourteen hours from twelve hours after we had requested experimenting with fewer hours of dialysis when the suffering was unbearable. This particular recollection frequently comes to mind because of its nature, and I shudder at the thought to this very day.

Transplant surgery was definitely his only interest. I should have assuredly known that in advance because I had seen Arthur's name on his blackboard under the heading of

"Transplant" together with other names. The concern to improve the lot of the dialysis patient in any way seemed to be totally lacking.

There was apparently nothing we could do except to bring up the matter of pure water to our own nephrologist. Lack of funds was his excuse. When our persistence proved to be unrelenting, he promised that budgeting for the pure water item would go on the following year's budget, because no funds were available.

But this doctor, too, had been an ardent transplant promoter. His telephone calls about available transplants had been fervent and frequent, sometimes bordering on the frantic. A rosy picture was painted for the future. We knew differently. We had seen too much happen to our friends on transplants to be optimistic.

Sometimes this doctor's argument would be that when the proposed transplant would eventually cease to function or in the event that it would not function at all, another transplant would be available. That, we certainly did not doubt. That which concerned us was that so many of our friends did not survive long enough to secure a second transplant. Oftentimes, the first kidney transplanted did not function normally. Implanting a new transplant is major surgery. Removing that kidney when rejected by the body is intervention. Implanting a second kidney in a greatly weakened body is further major surgery at maximum risk.

Strangely enough, the cost element was not a significant factor. From 1969 until 1973 the cost estimate for a transplant was often quoted to us as twenty thousand dollars. After being offered thirteen transplants, we requested that no further offers be made to us. If the day ever came when our minds would be changed, we would notify our doctor.

For our family, life would be supported by dialysis. Hopefully, there would be changes for the better. Why were obvious truths questioned? Clean water is preferable to contaminated water in every instance when cleanliness is to be achieved. Surely clean water without undesirable ingredients would mean a step forward for dialysis patients.

In January 1972, we moved as a family to another house a few blocks away from the parsonage that had been home to us for almost twelve years. We needed to be in this particular area near the university so our young people could attend classes and receive medical care.

The house was an older one with a gas radiant fireplace which gave a warm, friendly glow to the basement area. But the air seemed too dry in this large room away from the humidity provided by the water system in the furnace. Therefore, I took an empty, clear glass jar, filled it with water, and set it on the radiant. The water evaporated quickly; partial refilling was frequently necessary.

One day the jar had gone dry. Since it had become dull and soiled with a white, blotched coating, I decided to take it to the kitchen sink for a good washing. Soap and water would not remove the film. It was as if it were baked on from the heat of the radiant.

The truth was now crystal clear that water so contaminated with impurities of various kinds must be purified before being allowed to flow through the artificial kidney machines. How much residue would contaminate the bodies of kidney patients?

Late in January 1972, I telephoned the medical director of the University Hospital. To him our logic in regard to purified water seemed reasonable. He said, "I can see no reason why you can't have a little distilled water, Mrs. Olson."

The plan proposed to him was simply that Arthur be used as a single volunteer experimenter on a separate machine not attached to the central supply system.

The medical director's willingness to comply with this suggestion prompted our impulse to request three volunteers—our three young people to be on three separate machines individually supplied with distilled water. On the spur of the moment it occurred to me that there would be considerable difficulty in complying with such a demand at that time.

Common sense dictated that we be grateful for the unique privilege of using Arthur as a lone experimenter. It was sometime in February that Arthur's treatment on distilled water began. He had been on blood transfusions since December 1968.

On 8 March 1972, Arthur had his last blood transfusion. The distilled water had worked a miracle! Physical well-being increased with the rise in hemoglobin. We were ecstatic over the tremendous innovation.

Distilled water had the disadvantage of readily contaminating. Arthur suffered frequent severe infections. Therefore, we decided that deionized water would, in all probability, have greater virtue in regard to freedom from contamination.

On 12 July 1972, instead of a telephone call or a personal interview, I wrote a letter to the medical director. The promise of installing deionized water was subsequently to be fulfilled. The waiting period for the installation seemed terribly long. Carol and Joy's deterioration was visibly evident, and we knew by experience that help that seemed so near could be so far away. We telephoned frequently about more rapid progress. Every day counted. Life was at stake for so many, and for us the paramount concern was for our own two girls.

On 23 October 1972, came word that deionized water had been installed for the entire dialysis unit. I was at the dialysis unit the day the deionized water would be used in the water supply system for the first time. Before that period I had often worked with the young people during dialysis to ease the lot of our suffering family. A doctor who had opposed the introduction of purified water actually told me that the big day had come as he passed by me in the hall at the dialysis unit. I was jubilant. Our young people were ecstatic. We all sensed a surge of new hope, new progress, and new life that would revive the dialysis ward.

In the weeks and months that followed, the blood packs and blood transfusion equipment that had been so common a sight by so many beds gradually lessened in number. Carol was soon producing her own blood. For Joy, more time was required.

What a change had come to our household! Before purified water was introduced and survival had to be by means of contaminated tap water, Arthur had required a blood transfusion about every ten days. Carol had needed to have blood transfused weekly, and for Joy blood had been required every three, five or seven days. Life had been fast ebbing away for our Joy when purified, deionized water finally came to the rescue.

Our prayers had again been answered in a most marvelous way. And life had been sustained until this significant breakthrough, that had been so vigorously resisted, finally brought new life and hope.

To the Law Courts Building

The doctor came alone to Joy's room to ask for a bone biopsy during the time that she was on a metabolic study to determine the effectiveness of Dr. De Luca's experimental bone drug. Joy replied that Dr. De Luca had not made the bone biopsy a condition for the study. There were kidney patients who had been immobilized by such a biopsy, and that risk was one that our family was determined to avoid. The bone doctor swore and left.

The next day the same bone doctor returned and brought with him another doctor as his supporter. The bone doctor persisted in making disparaging remarks regarding Joy's reluctance to have a bone biopsy. The other doctor emphatically underlined each statement, as it were, in order to make Joy appear quite ridiculous. The bone doctor was like a ventriloquist having full control of his dummy doctor in a question and answer period. Two against one, the pressing proceeded, but Joy would not relent. She knew that what had happened by accident to others, could also happen to her. Furthermore, a second comparative bone study would be demanded later, but no mention was made of that customary procedure.

Then the bone doctor accompanied by the other doctor, took Joy in a wheelchair to see a man who was lying in bed on his stomach in another ward. That man had donated a cupful of bone marrow, the bone doctor said, and from Joy only a small quantity would be taken. The man who lay on his stomach praised the bone doctor and scoffed at Joy's reluctance. This time there were three against one.

Swearing all the while, the bone doctor belittled Joy for being hesitant and begrudging him a meager quantity of her bone marrow. Having suffered so intensely from bone pain, and having been in the operating room so frequently, he could not understand her unwillingness. If the new drug could relieve pain and permit her to walk with ease, that should be evidence enough for all concerned.

The bone doctor again insisted on her approval of a bone biopsy because, he said, he could not take her running, screaming and yelling. He needed consent. Joy was utterly weary of mind and body and she needed rest. In order to get rid of him temporarily, at least, she told him she would think about his demands. She intended to summon help and protection to preserve herself.

Joy, during the time of the metabolic study, was being dialyzed in isolation because she was supposed to have a positive Australian antigen. Her chart went with her from her ward to the isolation ward. On examining her chart, she discovered the doctor's handwritten comment that Joy would be having a bone biopsy as soon as she signed her consent. For the doctor it was just a matter of time. The delay caused by her refusal was an aggravation that would be duly overcome. Next morning the bone doctor again made his appearance for the same purpose. Joy, again, said she would think about his request in order to lengthen her time. The opportunity came for her to telephone home to plead for direct help and intervention because there would obviously be no end to the insistent pressuring of this angry, profane doctor. Joy complained that the emotional stress had completely exhausted her both mentally and physically, and she was at the point of despair.

The news angered me. Why should a doctor force more suffering upon one who had suffered so much, especially when a very real risk was involved? She had declined for a good reason. She surely had the right to determine what should be done to her body. Why did he not respect her wishes?

It was, I remember, with considerable difficulty that I finally located him by telephone. I told him that we definitely disapproved of his series of persistent tactics, that Joy's wishes must be respected and that she be, henceforth, left alone and not subjected to such incessant badgering. His reaction seemed to be that a bigger and an older person must be dispatched with a louder, longer, and stronger volley of abuse. It was evident that he was not accustomed to opposition and that he would not readily accept defeat. But, defeated he was, and that in five emphatic words: "There will be no biopsy."

To the Law Courts Building I went, after having received permission to have an interview with a prominent personage who was a member of the Kidney Foundation. It seemed likely that he would be willing to advise our young bone doctor privately and put him on a better course of conduct.

Never before had I been in the Law Courts Building. The judge sat behind his desk in this office-like room, and a man in uniform made a formal introduction to his honour, the judge. I was ushered into a sort of private boxed-off area at a good distance but within easy hearing range.

"And what have I gotten myself into this time?" I wondered to myself. I wasn't at complete ease, to say the least. I had not expected the judge to be dressed in his courtly navy uniform in readiness for his appointed sitting on the bench that afternoon. I noticed the handsome flared cuffs on his coat and scanned his entire apparel. Two buttons were very obviously missing. That amused me and served to settle me down. He was, after all, very ordinary indeed.

My concerns about informed consent were aired quite freely and the sins of the young bone doctor were duly exposed. It seemed that this man could and would privately attend to these grave matters in his own way and direct the offender onto a straighter and narrower path. In fact, as the following months and years passed we were no longer subjected to such harassment by him.

Another doctor, who had also profited by similar help from a senior doctor, told our son that the Kidney Foundation would henceforth be well-staffed by lawyers insofar as possible. That precaution, he ventured, would ensure cheap legal fees and protection against kidney patients who might endeavor to engage in lawsuits to maintain or regain their rights, or to determine their full rights.

The Law Courts episode served to expose the errors of the kidney dialysis system to one more significant person. There was a change, as far as we were concerned, in the care given us by two doctors. Informed consent was coming into its own. The fact that the consent must be willing and not forced or manipulated was a subtle side issue that needed to be fully resolved.

Arthur and I Respond to Dialysis—1975

Machine Progress

Times of crises brought alternatives in treatment that proved to be of immeasurable help to our physical well-being. Arthur's liver infection of 1970 was no exception. Because of the need for isolation technique, his doctor ordered him on peritoneal dialysis. Although acknowledging the need for isolation, Arthur would not submit to this form of treatment which he knew would require surgery and be time-consuming and uncomfortable. He was firm in his conviction that he would not suffer physically in any way save the suffering that was inevitable on the artificial kidney machine. A furious doctor told my mother he wished Arthur would die and that he should have ordered the treatment without saying anything.

A new artificial kidney machine offered promise of halving the length of time on dialysis. Six hours of treatment on this Travenol Coil machine accomplished the work of twelve hours of terrible discomfort and fatigue on the Kiil machine. This was truly wonderful and provided us with the possibility of a more promising future.

We asked, then implored our doctors to purchase the Travenol Coil machine. They reminded us of the tight budget. It was difficult to accept that the relatively small amount of money needed to purchase this machine stood between Arthur and a new lease on life. It soon came to our attention that one Travenol machine was "collecting dust in a closet." Because our unit was a Kiil unit, no other machines were to be used. So said the director of the kidney unit.

My father asked the director of the kidney unit if the purpose of the artificial kidney machine program was to provide the chronic renal failure patient with the best life possible and alleviate suffering. To this the director replied, "Kidney patients must learn to suffer." Defeated, my father, a minister, continued to pray to our Heavenly Father that He would open the hearts of these men of influence to see our need and bring to us this machine that promised a better life.

The medical director of our hospital asked to see my father together with the director of the kidney unit. My father presented our case; and happily for us, the medical director had the compassion to let Arthur begin treatment on a Travenol Coil machine. It was a day for rejoicing in our household.

My first hemodialysis experience was two hours on the Kiil, the second was four hours, the third was to be eight hours. Standard treatment at this time was three eight-hour hemodialysis sessions per week. However, after four and one-half hours of the eight hour shift, I begged to be taken off hemodialysis because of a severe reaction which left me in a state of physical collapse. Joy had the same experience. It was obvious we would not survive long if this physical trauma continued.

My mother approached the director of the kidney unit regarding the policy of standard hours of treatment. It seemed common sense that a person who weighed ninety kilograms would need longer hemodialysis than one who weighed forty-five kilograms. We believed the individual should be assessed for length of hemodialysis through the evaluation of blood results, weight, and diet, taking into account related factors such as the flow-rate of blood through the dialyzer and the condition of the dialysis access.

Mother promised she would accept moral and legal responsibility for any harm that resulted from this approach to hemodialysis care. Acknowledging that we could not be forced to take the prescribed treatment, the amused doctor let her have her way. The concept of too much dialysis proved credible in the place of the concept that the longer the dialysis, the better, which had caused so much suffering for so many. Unfortunately, this benefit won for ourselves was a long time in coming for others.

Even with fewer hours of hemodialysis, Joy, who is tiny, continued to suffer because the volume of blood circulating outside the body during hemodialysis strained her heart. We asked the director of the kidney unit if a machine requiring less volume was available. The introduction of the Travenol Coil at the unit had opened the way for the experimental use of other dialyzers. The director of the unit suggested the Gambro, a series of compact disposable dialyzers with approximately the volume of the Kiil and more efficient filtration rate resulting in fewer hours of hemodialysis. The Gambro was so successful in terms of patient comfort and well-being on and between hemodialysis that the Kiil became only a bad memory.

Following the success of the Gambro, various models of Cordis-Dows were tried. The Dow is also a compact disposable dialyzer which combines the features of increased surface area with small volume for rapid filtration. I agreed to try the Dow in hopes of regulating my high serum potassium/low sodium levels which were a problem for me on the Kiil and Gambro. This the Dow accomplished and I no longer lived under the constant threat of heart arrest caused by potassium-sodium imbalance.

Blood

Even with the improvements in dialysis, a serious problem remained: the inability of our bodies to produce hemoglobin (the oxygen-carrying pigment of the blood). I required a blood transfusion once weekly; Arthur needed one approximately every ten days; Joy, every three or four days. Standard treatment required that the patient receive two units of blood each time a transfusion was needed. Arthur asked that one transfusion be given because he endured frequent reactions as he developed antibodies in response to multiple transfusions. Two doctors rejected the proposal, one finally agreed. One transfusion proved to be as effective as two and this procedure was incorporated in place of the other.

Once an intern came to see me when I was an in-patient after I had needed an emergency transfusion. He said I had caused quite a stir with my low hemoglobin and he asked me if I knew what the reading was. I told him that it had been 3.0, a weekly experience for me. He scoffed, saying that it was impossible for anyone to live with a hemoglobin below 5.0. I smiled to myself as he left. He was right. One couldn't live but one could exist.

Sometimes I wondered where reality was. I had promised myself I would center my life in real life pursuits, yet my involvement at the university seemed unreal. I walked down the halls with my heart thumping in my head, breathing slowly and deeply to avoid gasping for air. My lungs and muscles ached, I was wrapped in fatigue. The make-up I wore was a mask—under its artificial glow, I looked pale and felt lifeless. On one occasion in particular, the separateness of our lives jarred me when a group of students asked, "And what did you do on the weekend?" I wondered what I should tell them. That I was caught in the hopeless cycle of Friday blood transfusions? That I had had another reaction on hemodialysis? That another friend had died? That at the moment I was leaning against the wall to keep my knees from buckling underneath me? I smiled in reply. It was just as well. Already they were laughing about another incident.

Blood Water

One day my mother noticed the glass jar that had held tap water which had evaporated. A heavy white deposit was left in the jar. She wondered what effect this water would have on our blood during the long periods of hemodialysis. The thought occurred that an improvement might be to use distilled or deionized water instead of tap water to mix with and dilute the dialysate (the cleaning fluid) that cleanses the blood of its impurities as it travels through the artificial kidney machine.

Our doctors were unwilling to try this, maintaining that there was no proof for such a practise; however, they were willing to risk a transplant or a splenectomy. The spleen was enlarging and becoming overactive in the destruction of red blood cells due to constant blood transfusions. This enlarged spleen therefore becomes a secondary cause of low hemoglobin. Removal of the spleen does not remedy the initial cause of low hemoglobin.

We took our case to the medical director of the hospital who stated, "I can't see why you can't have a little distilled water." In February 1972, Arthur began using distilled water in his treatments. Two months later, he discontinued blood transfusions and never required one since. Plagued with a deteriorating skeletal system, the increased hemoglobin gave Arthur the needed energy to move about with the aid of artificial supports instead of being completely confined to a wheelchair. Also, increased energy resulted in greater visual capability because Arthur's damaged eyes did not tire so easily. No longer did he require another's blood. To a limited degree, Arthur experienced independence and self-sufficiency even though he was still tied to the machine.

Arthur was freed from the prison of anemia. Joy and I were desperate for release. Our family petitioned doctors and administrators for months arguing in favor of deionized water. The alternative that was becoming a common part of hemodialysis care was the splenectomy. I noted the dubious results of the surgery as some spleenless patients stabilized at hemoglobins of 4.0. A friend who suffered as we did was told there was no scientific proof for the Olsons' belief in deionized water even though Arthur was no longer on blood transfusions. It was unlikely the water would be pumped into the unit. Our good friend told us he was desperate. He had the spleenectomy and died soon afterward. Another friend took the transplant route to escape transfusions. She, too, was desperate for a satisfying life and she was full of hope for the future following her wedding engagement. She too died.

But some of us waited in hope, longing for the day of fulfillment. In sorrow and frustation we waited—writing, telephoning, interviewing, struggling through the passing days. Eight months we waited for the deionized or distilled water to be piped into the unit. And then, the miracle. Suddenly, I needed a transfusion only once a month, then once in two months, then never again. My hemoglobin had become self-maintained at 5.0; within myself was the pulse-beat of life. Purified water provided ourselves and our friends with a new lease on life.

New Bone, New Life

Evident in our familial kidney ailment was a debilitating bone disease causing deformity and severe bone pain. When Arthur began hemodialysis, he was already experiencing bone pain in joints and ribs. As the first few years on the kidney machine progressed, the bone pain steadily worsened and the deformity increased. His legs began to bend at the knees, his ribs became barrel-shaped, and his head bones were sinking. He was becoming a cripple.

Two parathyroidectomy operations, increased calcium in the dialysate, and increased amounts of vitamin D did nothing to help Arthur's situation. Walking very short distances became possible only with the aid of artificial supports such as crutches and full-length leg braces. Longer distances were possible only with the aid of a wheelchair. Mother pushed his wheelchair to get to classes at the university because his bones were too weak and painful to even push the wheelchair wheels, again and again.

In the fall of 1971 the director of the kidney unit told Arthur that nothing more could be done for his deteriorating skeletal system, and that his only hope was a kidney transplant. Arthur was aware that research was being carried out in the area of producing a kidney metabolite of vitamin D which is necessary for the normal bone-building process. Since he lacked the necessary kidney function to produce this metabolite of vitamin D, it seemed to be a possibility for his problem. We asked for the name of someone in this area of research and were referred to Dr. H. F. DeLuca of the University of Wisconsin-Madison. We related to Dr. DeLuca our immediate need; he replied that November, telling us a liver metabolite was available and that his Department of Biochemistry had theoretically conceived of an active kidney metabolite of vitamin D. In a matter of time he would have enough for Arthur to begin on a long-term treatment.

Our doctors were to gain the acceptance of the Food and Drug Administration in both the United States and Canada before the drug would be brought in. They showed even less enthusiasm or interest in bringing this drug than they had for the purified water experiment. Disinterest and denials that this vitamin D compound was being made added to the frustration. At one time we sent copies of Dr. DeLuca's initial letter to our own doctors in the hope that someone would take up this cause. This hope, too, was frustrated. After many months the liver metabolite (25 hydroxy) came. Dr. DeLuca during this time was busy making enough of the 1,25 compound to begin Arthur on a long-term treatment.

It was a glorious day when Arthur went into the hospital to begin treatment on a metabolic study, the purpose of which was to measure the ability of the compound to absorb calcium from the intestine and put it into the blood stream for use in bone restoration. The planned nine-week study was so successful that after seven weeks the study was terminated. During this time bone pain lessened to the degree that he could move with ease when not bearing weight on his bones. Lying on what used to be cracked ribs, grasping with his hands, eased as time moved on.

By August of 1974, eight months later, Arthur had literally thrown away his crutches, braces, and his wheelchair for the last time. To move with ease, walk with ease, and conduct music with ease had become a part of his life. It is difficult to put into words the freedom he now enjoyed and the thankfulness in his heart towards Dr. DeLuca and God who had raised him up to newness of life. That time he could honestly say that he had had two lifelines—the artificial kidney machine and the 1,25 dihydroxycholecalciferol vitamin D3. Without the artificial kidney machine he would no longer know life; and without the 1,25 compound, life would be mere existence.

Our family rejoiced together at the miraculous restoration of Arthur's skeletal system. His bones had been sunken, deformed. His face had registered the gnawing pain. Up from the wheelchair he stood, walked, ran. We praised God.

In the fall of 1974, it appeared that Arthur's past might become my future. I was experiencing early signs of bone deterioration. My shoulder bones were bending and I was in danger of falling because of weak ankles. The 1,25 was produced experimentally in small quantities but its synthetic analogue, 1 alpha, was more easily made and, therefore, more readily available in good supply. When I asked the new director of the kidney unit for this drug to prevent the disease from progressing, and recoup the damage it had done, I was told, "No bone biopsy, no drug."

Although a bone biopsy is a painful procedure, it is valuable only as a statistical device which indicates the type of bone disease and its stage of progression. Another statistical device is the densitometer, which measures the bone density using numerical and graphic equivalents. Each result is relative to the others, as a positive or negative trend is indicated. The densinometer looks like x-ray equipment and is administered similarly without discomfort to the patient.

I refused to undergo the bone biopsy because it was presented to me as a threat and because I rebelled against needless suffering. The doctors were adamant. My family was adamant. My mother wrote a circular letter to hospital administrators, Food and Drug administrators, a major drug company in the United States, two Canadian kidney specialists and Dr. H. F. DeLuca who made the vitamin D compound. This letter stressed my immediate need for the compound as a preventive medicine and the similar need of countless people with kidney failure suffering from bone deterioration. Finally the phone call came. I was promised the 1 alpha, no strings attached.

A month later I began 1 alpha therapy. My ankles stopped troubling me. More slowly, my skeletal frame has straightened. I am thankful to the men whose compassion matched their power to bring the 1 alpha to me.

Protection from Medicine

Different dialyzers, individualized procedures, improvements in treatments were all changes—some obvious and some not so obvious—that have proved to have beneficial effects. Drastic changes in our quality of life and therefore, our longevity were due to benefits that had been obtained either by ourselves on our own, or by persistent argument with doctors, or by going to medical personnel and authorities beyond our doctors.

Why the opposition to these changes by our doctors? The grim reality was that the renal program at the University Hospital was research-oriented. Supported by million-dollar grants, research directly and indirectly affected and dictated what happened in the care and treatment of the hemodialysis patients at our kidney unit. Research is a necessity of medical science and therefore has its place in the relatively new field of chronic and acute renal failure care. However, when this research interferes with the implementation of treatment and procedures that are beneficial to the long-term hemodialysis patient, it must be questioned.

Our family realized long ago that research will never be removed from our kidney unit. We, therefore, have attempted to move through the hierarchy of the University Hospital in our attempt to improve the quality of our lives and the lives of other patients, and to protect ourselves from the inherent dangers of research-oriented medical practices.

Patient Education for Individual Care

Access from the patient's artery and vein to the arterial and venous lines of the artificial kidney machine is necessary for hemodialysis treatment. There are two basic connections possible: the cannula and the fistula. The cannula consists of two tubes surgically inserted in an artery and a vein in a limb. These two tubes remain with one at all times so that the cannula is actually an extension of the body's artery and vein system. The fistula consists of an arm artery and vein which are surgically joined. Needles are used to connect the artery and vein to the arterial and venous lines of the machine. In order to accept the machine as a part of our lives, we had to also accept the responsibility of caring for the cannula—cleaning, bandaging. To accept the fistula or a

fistula-related connection as our life-line requires the acceptance of needles with every hemodialysis treatment and the
possibility of long periods of bleeding from the needle sites
after hemodialysis treatments.

Although various problems such as clotting and infections
have plagued us at times, the three of us are very thankful
that we had been spared needles in our arms for the hemodialysis treatments duration. There are others on dialysis
with fistulas who are thankful they are spared the problems
which occur with cannulas.

Patients going on the machine need to be truthfully told
the pros and cons of both the cannula and the fistula (and
fistula-related connections) in order to make the choice that
is right for them. Since this is a personal life-line, the
individual's choice must be respected. Too often one sided
arguments are presented by kidney unit doctors according
to their preference.

Informed Consent for Individual Care

Joy suffered from low hemoglobin long after the rest of
us had self-maintained hemoglobins. The doctors pressed her
to try testosterone, a male hormone which has the possible
side-effect of raising hemoglobin. But other possible effects
are cancer, the lowering of the voice, and the appearance of
facial hair and general masculinity. Joy refused, maintaining
that testosterone's disadvantages outweighed its possible
advantage.

Before the following hemodialysis treatment, she read the
doctor's order on her chart for an injection of the hormone—
one c.c. in each buttock. Although Joy had refused, pressure
was exerted for months each time Joy had problems with a
low hemoglobin. She insisted she had the right to know and
to say no. The trauma experienced by Joy in her attempts
to protect herself from this constant pressure was great.

Informed consent provides us with the protection and
responsibility necessary to live the most self-satisfying and
personally acceptable life with chronic renal failure, and
guarantees a certain degree of individual care. But the system

at the kidney unit did not foster individual care. A policy of patient independence was enforced with rigor which had each patient rinse and set up his machine before hemodialysis treatments. No matter the strain of real life pursuits, hemoglobin level, bone deterioration, or whatever, this time-consuming task was part and parcel of life on the kidney machine.

We acknowledged the need to understand dialysis but could not see the logic of this mechanical task as proof of our independence and acceptance of dialysis. We were fulfilling our career goals in life which was proof enough of our acceptance and independence.

Part way through 1973, Joy was wearing out physically, mentally, and emotionally from her university load because of very low hemoglobin and severe bone deterioration. She found it increasingly difficult to come into the kidney unit after a day's work and attempt to do her assigned task with a cannula in one arm and a bone fracture in the other. Difficult, too, was rinsing the machine while staff stood around and watched. Some nurses wanted to help. Approached many times, Joy's doctor seemed to understand Joy's immediate need and promised that her machine would be rinsed for her; however, no change came.

It would take too long to tell of the many meetings, panel examinations, interviews with administrators and petitions. But improvements finally were made. The nursing staff increased in number to the point that oftentimes there were more nurses than patients at the unit. The cleanliness of the physical plant of the unit was much improved. No nurse put a patient on or off the machine without gloves. Doctors were a little more regular in their rounds to see us at the kidney unit which had previously been a hit and miss affair.

Illness is Personal

Our doctors made a change in treatment that was very worthwhile; three treatments a week instead of the previous two. However, the problem of too much hemodialysis became apparent. Because the three of us were responsible for the number of hours of treatment we took, it was necessary for us to know and understand our monthly bloodwork results which register the effectiveness of our treatments in removing impurities from the blood.

The director of the unit was very reluctant to do this and three times gave permission and then denied it. Finally, consent was given us to evaluate our monthly bloodwork results. With the introduction of a variety of kidney machines at our kidney unit and number of hours of treatment dictated by monthly bloodwork results for the shortest hemodialysis possible, the three of us enjoyed a measure of individual care.

At one time, for example, I required salt but needed to carefully watch my potassium intake. Joy enjoyed more potassium foods but restricted sodium intake. Arthur used more salt than Joy, but much less than I and could have as much potassium food as Joy. Two of us had very little fluid intake. These restrictions allowed Joy, who weighed 33 kilograms to be treated on a Gambro 17 Micron dialyzer for three hours each time. Arthur, weighing 50 kilograms and I, weighing 45 kilograms, were treated on the Cordis Dow dialyzer for three and three-quarter hours and three and one-half hours respectively.

The fewest hours of hemodialysis possible that guarantee efficient bloodwork; the fewest drugs and smallest doses needed to maintain whatever balance that does not result from diet or hemodialysis (vitamins and phosphate binders only, if possible); the least blood taken at any time to ensure the highest hemoglobin possible; the least amount of anti-coagulant (used on hemodialysis to avoid clotting of blood) to ensure freedom from bruising and bleeding between treatments; restricted fluid intake for the least amount of negative pressure applied while on hemodialysis (needed to remove excess fluid gain from our blood): all are examples of how we have tried to make our lives on dialysis the least traumatic possible. Such procedures have aided our relative physical well-being.

CHAPTER 3

THE QUESTION OF TECHNOLOGY

The more fundamental a question, the more it
demands that the self-understanding of the
question be itself examined and interpreted.

—David C. Hoy

Children of Technology

All of humanity are children of technology. All through
history, we make our self technologically; what else could we
make? The peasant's life is harnessed to the plow he made.
The shepherd's life is managed with the staff he made. Our
life, too, is conjoined to the tools we inherit and invent. And
these tools that we make, ever more diverse and complex, re-
make us.

All our making empties us; our life is poured into the
works of our hands. We are dis-spirited; technology is the
spirit of the age, our immortal body. The ruins of other
civilizations are tributes to their makers, effigies of the
human will to immortality. But we pioneer the making of
our self in our corporeal image—the respirator, the artificial
kidney machine—life after death on earth. So the world and
everything in it, including our self, appears as though we
made it. We are set apart from technology's other children:
we are technology's chosen people. We see a use for everything.
We see nothing more than use-value in anything. So we cling
to what we have made, even the tools of our own destruction,
and we believe in what we can make. Technology is us. What
will become of us? Dr. Chayatte, a medical doctor on dialysis,

wrote this poem "To my fellow patients in the certain knowledge that life is more than survival."

> I am victim, I am victor,
> For death will win its waiting game.
> Momentarily I have tricked her
> Fanned life's fading flame.
>
> But life is worthwhile living,
> Uncertain day to day
> When you can be doing, giving,
> When the world heeds what you say.
>
> Leave me without purpose;
> Take my self-esteem;
> As well to leave me lifeless
> Than only alive on a machine.[1]

Many of technology's chosen people have already fled, like chirping lemmings, into the abyss. Some of us stopped at the edge of the cliff. We have re-turned. We come, raving fluently like Nietzsche's madman, "Whither is God... We have killed him—you and I."[2] We must speak this way: we have seen the abyss. And, we come, speaking haltingly, our words breaking under the awesome silence of each sacred breath. We must speak this way: we have seen the "bright morning star."[3] Either way, we come with empty hands. We offer our being— the abyss and the star, ancient measure of the measure of technology.

Dialysis

I am one of technology's chosen people: my life is maintained by dialysis. Dialysis is the technology for cleansing the blood when kidneys die. Is dialysis only this? More than this? Even when we consider dialysis strictly as a relationship with a machine, dialysis is already us. Three people describe their dialysis experiences:

> I'm only 32 years old. Yet, in terms of dialysis, I'm a grand-father. At least, that's the way I feel when I look back on the fourteen years I've been friends with a kidney machine.[4]

> I could never take a vacation from the machine I married
> till death do us part.[5]

> The journey through the years with technology is a human
> journey—dependence on the machine, rebellion from the
> machine, oneness with the machine.[6]

But dialysis is not strictly a relationship with a machine.
Dialysis is a relationship with others—doctors, nurses, family,
friends. And through all this, dialysis is a relationship with
life.
  Recollection of 1972:

> I asked the doctor for an innovation which would make life
> easier.
> "You're never satisfied," he said. "If I give you what you
> ask for, you'll ask for something more."
> I agreed.
> "But this is artificial life support!" he said. "What do you
> want out of it anyway?"
> "Everything."
> He stared at me for a moment, then hurried away.
> That evening, I repeated to myself, "Everything. I want
> everything."

> I asked for all things that I might enjoy life.
> I was given life that I might enjoy all things.[7]

Year by year, doctor and patient encounter each other. Yet
each life is hidden from the other behind tests, statistics,
protocol; separated from the other by the technology that
brings us together:

> The nature and importance of our relationship to one
> another is a core issue in every society, system of ethics,
> and religion. Dialysis and transplantation have re-empha-
> sized how central it is to medicine as well. This has occurred
> in a period of generalized crisis over whether and how an
> advanced modern society like our own can achieve a more
> trusting, intimate, inclusive, and transcendent form of
> solidarity.[8]

The crisis: we have forgotten how to listen and to speak with each other. But *what* have we forgotten?

The Meaning of Speaking and Listening

The ancient Greek theorist, Heraclitus (6th century, B.C.),[9] believed that speech is essentially a moral responsibility of community members. The ancient Greek responsibility for community was called forth in the image and in the activity of caring for the hearth-fire; the hearth-fire which provided warmth and togetherness for the members of the family. Caring for the hearth-fire was a caring for the community, the collective family. This life the ancient Greeks called logos. So logos was not inherent in any fire but in their care and use of the fire they kept at the center of their dwellings, at the center of their lives, in the hearth. Care transformed the fire and those who tended, used, and shared it. So, logos is the calling together of community (the fire that gathers individuals together in care for each other) and the community that is called (those who are gathered in care for the fire).

The most profound attunement to logos is shown when we near the fire and are scarred by it for the good of another. This is our rational character; "the verb, *charassein* (Gk), from which character is derived, means 'to scratch,' 'to scar,' or otherwise mark. Those, then, who have suffered the ordeal of nearing logos bear the scar of rationality."[10] We still speak of a face having character. Character is born of care: one who cares (Gothic from Gk. *kara*, 'sorrow')[11] sorrows for another, bears the sorrow of another. We say that the face having character is lined with care.[12] Care as the rationality (L. *ratio*, 'reason')[13] of community life was given to the ancient Greeks as the possibility they must thoughtfully choose for community life to continue. At the same time, the rationality of care was given before thought, in self-forgetfulness at this moment, as when loving parents respond to the needs of their infant son or daughter, often before the child cries. To belong to logos is to belong to each other: "listening not to me [the speaker] but to the logos it is wise to agree that all things are one."[14]

To dialogue is to speak and listen to each other in the light of logos. To speak is to (re)direct conversation towards logos as that which shows logos. To listen is to hear not merely the speaker but rather to "sustain yourself in hearkening attunement [to logos]."[15] So, to understand something in the light of logos is to presuppose an attitude of care for it and for the community that shines through speech and silence. An attitude of care is both hidden and revealed in commonly used medical terms such as cardiology, nephrology, neurology. The suffix of each of these terms derives from logos. Therefore, cardiology means to speak about—care for—the heart in a way that listens to—cares for—the meaning of the heart in the life of a human being, in the life of a community.

Logos joins our separate lives into a collective endeavor by calling each one to a personal commitment to care for the good of each one. "It is not in being attentive to the speeches of men, but in heeding our calling, that we achieve the sort of agreement that collects all things."[16] For example, 'hospitality' began as an expression of the ancient Greeks' personal and community commitment to care for wayfaring strangers.[18] The stranger was welcomed as a friend would be welcomed. Each house was built with a room (Gk. *hospitalia* or *hospitalium*) for the stranger. In this way, the stranger was provided for in the physical structure of the community. But the stranger was truly a guest in the home—the heads of the household became the host (Gk. *hospis*) and hostess (Gk. *hospita*) as they invited the guest to share the family meal. The ancient Romans provided for strangers in a similar manner. Private hospitality gradually extended to public hospitality but 'hospital' derives not from its public nature but from a reference to the guest (L. *hospitalis*). An ancient Greek and Roman tradition, *tessera hospitalis*, reveals the bond that developed between the stranger-guest and the hosting family. It was a medallion which guest and host divided and kept as a token of lasting friendship, not only during the lives of the friends but during the lives of their descendants. (The sign of a broken friendship was the breaking of one's part of the *tessera hospitalis*.) Provision for the stranger was the logos of community life.

What can a human science researcher in our technological society learn from Heraclitus about "heeding our calling"?

Many human science researchers forget their calling—forget their indebtedness to logos for illumining the things which science analyzes. Heraclitus warns that logos "escapes men's notice because of their infidelity."[18] Infidelity to logos results in scientific investigation which is alienated from community life. Perhaps doctors and patients have forgotten how to listen and to speak with each other because we have forgotten logos, our collective life; we have forgotten logos, our rational character.

CHAPTER 4

THE QUESTION OF UNDERSTANDING

By thinking comes to mind the longings of my heart.

—Ghada Daabous

Can We Understand?

The ancient Greek theorist, Heraclitus, was certain that his message, "All is one," belonged to the origin of community. The truth of the ancient Greek sense of certainty shines through history in the example of the peasant whose life is harnessed to the plough he made. This sense of certainty is called forth by the rhythm of seedtime and harvest, cold and heat; grain in abundance, grain wanting; child born, child dying. The life of the peasant is the soil—from dawn to dusk, from dust to dust. Yet a question wells up through the certainty of the life called forth for and by the peasant's life: "Is there more to life than this?" The ancient Greek theorist knew this question, the question that called forth theorizing. "Is there more to life?" is another way of asking, "What belongs to logos, to our community, to each other?"

Technology's chosen people are certain only of the resource-fullness of everything. The meaning of anything is only its use to us. This is our life.[1] But we are exhausting the resourcefulness of everything, and still the grain is wanting, still the children die. Is there more to life for us?

To search through the question, "Is there more to life for us?" we must suspend—"bracket"[2]—our certainty that everything is only resourceful so that we might experience

65

life anew. Bracketing our technological certainty is the
starting point for this inquiry.

Hermeneutic Phenomenology

> 'Phenomenology' is a name which is mainly used to
> designate a movement in the social and human sciences
> which has as its primary objective the direct investigation
> and description of phenomena as consciously (i.e., pre-
> theoretically) experienced.[3]

> Hermeneutics may be defined as the science of interpre-
> tation, or as the phenomenology of social understanding.[4]

Hermeneutic phenomenology is the dialectical understanding, "All is one." On the one hand, we are woven into
the fabric of life. Merleau-Ponty expresses this understanding
of experience when he writes, "he who sees cannot possess
the visible unless he is possessed by it, unless he is of it."[5]
On the other hand, "Understanding begins," writes Gadamer,
"when something addresses us."[6] Something addresses us
when it lifts itself out of the pattern in the fabric of everyday
life and "shows itself in itself."[7] This understanding of
dialectic is exemplified by van Manen, who writes that the
presence of children calls us to choose teaching as a way of
life which "orients us to the flesh of the world, as Merleau-
Ponty poetized, to the intertwining, where I am not with the
child, not in the world, but where I am the child, the world."[8]
"Intertwining" is possible because our experience of childhood
addresses us in the person of each child we meet. Through
the oneness of the intertwining we experience more deeply
our separateness, as when a child does not understand the
instruction we had planned specifically for her. We respond
in a manner called teaching when we experience the child's
misunderstanding and so, are enabled to lead the child out.
Our intertwining attunes us to our separateness; our
separateness enables our intertwining.

This dialectic is further exemplified by our experience of
language. We say, "The sun is setting," though our day is
setting and the sun is fixed. The silence of a day that is spent

rests in this idiom as does the promise, "Tomorrow is another day." Language is not so much a resource for speaking (a vocabulary list) as a source for speaking (a well-spring). Each day brings new experience that is centuries old. As we transform the day into our life by the way we live, so we transform the experience into its meaning by the way we speak. The words on the vocabulary list become a well-spring of meaning for us. This unique experience of the day and its words opens up to us a dimension of language which hearkens back to centuries old communal experience, while welcoming the not-yet-experienced. We wait for language, and language waits for us.

We live this dialectic when we express our response to the questions life addresses to us moment by moment with speech and silence, labor and rest, worship and praise. And yes, with research. Illness addresses us in this research. How can we express our response to illness?

Expressing Our Response to Illness

There are two main ways of expressing our response to illness. One way is to try to control illness technologically by making it predictable. A vehicle of technological control is explanation which puts things in order. For example, we explain the progression of a disease and the effects of a medical intervention. When we explain, we stand apart from the phenomenon and observe the order. Explanation has provided answers to many problems, yet explanation does not help us to know the question, "Is there more to life for us?"

The finality of explanation belies the mystery of the intertwining and our participation in this mystery: through all our experiences, each of us is uniquely enmeshed in the fabric of life. For example, two people with the 'same' disease respond differently to the 'same' medical intervention. Description, rather than explanation, 'speaks' our experience of illness. When we describe, we do not invest the phenomenon with meaning. We open ourselves up to the idea which inhabits the phenomenon, the idea which makes the experience of the phenomenon intelligible to us. "An idea," writes

Proust, "is not the contrary of the sensible [the phenomenon],"
it is "its lining and its depth."[9] W. H. Auden shows that the
idea comes to us in visible, tangible experience in his poetic
description of what it is like to be in a surgical ward.

> They are and suffer; that is all they do;
> A bandage hides the place where each is living,
> His knowledge of the world restricted to
> The treatment that the instruments are giving.
>
> And lie apart like epochs from each other—
> Truth in their sense is how much they can bear;
> It is not talk like ours, but groans they smother—
> And are remote as plants; we stand elsewhere.
>
> For who when healthy can become a foot?
> Even a scratch we can't recall when cured,
> But are boist'rous in a moment and believe
>
> In the common world of the uninjured, and cannot
> Imagine isolation. Only happiness is shared,
> And anger, and the idea of love.[10]

In contrast to an explanation concerning post-surgical
trauma, Auden's poem opens up a world of shared experience.
We participate in the truth of the poem: the silence that gives
voice to each word, each phrase, is our silence, our "mute
experience."[11] As we enter into dialogue with Auden's poem,
we begin to speak the silence of our experience. "For who
when healthy can become a foot?" The whole body, a foot.
The whole foot, pain. There is no other world. I am the foot-
in-pain, waiting for the next dose that will move this foot,
this pain, out there, while I remain here, still conscious that
a foot-in-pain hurts somewhere. My only thought, a prayer
that this dose will last the four hours until the next dose. My
religion, my time—my life—bound up in the foot-in-pain, here
or there. Lord, keep it out there. The mute experience of the
foot-in-pain that pre-dates the reading of the poem becomes
articulate when we read the poem. As the poem remembers
in us our solitary experience, it confirms in us our solidarity

with our community. Our interpretation of the poem is the poem's interpretation of us.

As the poem articulates for us and in us an experience of surgery, the poem asks for continued reflection in its light, and we become ready to read the poem though we may never see it in print again. In this way, we stand under the poem that understands us. Hunsberger writes, "When a reader gains insight and a broader, clearer vision, and is able to see the patterns and the wholeness, that understanding becomes a part of who the reader is and how that reader relates to others."[13] We learn to live. Merleau-Ponty writes, "Life becomes ideas and ideas return to life."[13] Phenomenology expresses this "reversibility" ("always imminent though never realized in fact")[14] through dialogue.

Experience as Dialogue

We search for the future through dialogue with what is past. We do not recall events that are over. Rather, our experience lives in us, making us what we are.[15] An experience is a moment in which what belongs to logos 'speaks.' Gadamer writes,

> Experience is a matter of multisided disillusionment based on expectation; only in this way is experience acquired. The fact that experience is preeminently painful and unpleasant does not really color experience black, it lets us see into the inner nature of experience.[16]

Something is not as we had expected. For example, we expect to use specific tools to facilitate our daily existence. Tools are transparent in use, extensions of ourselves.[17] The hammer exists for us in the pounding of the nail. Though we grip the handle of a hammer, we feel the clang of its head on a nail. But suppose we expect to use a hammer and find it broken. "Breakdown," writes Heidegger, "momentarily lights up the being of tool as tool."[18] Breakdown asks for dialogue. Similarly, our own breaking asks us what wholeness is. The foot that is healthy does not question us nor do we question it; we simply use it to walk and rest. The loss of this foot—injured or amputated—changes us. There is truth here, which the walking foot, the resting foot, could not teach us. There is pain here, the pain of brokenness. This pain, Gadamer calls the "inner nature" of experience.

Gustave Thibon brings to speech the pain of past and present experience in dialectic with hope for the future. Our future is our heritage.

> You feel you are hedged in; you dream of escape. Do not run or fly away in order to get free: rather dig in the narrow place which has been given you; you will find God there and everything. God does not float on your horizon, he sleeps in your substance. Vanity runs, love digs.[19]

"Vanity runs, love digs." So we repair our broken tools, preparing a future for ourselves as we use them. Our suffering and rejoicing in our work is hope in action. In this resoluteness of hope shines the promise of our future—*our* future because we live in community. To live in community means to speak and listen to each other. The individual responds to the question of the other, ready to give his world in speech and silence, ready to listen to—to welcome—the other who shines forth in her speech and silence.[20]

A personal-communal tradition streams through each individual. The voice of each individual is "bound to the mass of [his] own life as is the voice of no one else."[21] Each individual speaks from experience. Speaking from experience is "not like the butter on the bread;" it is "the expression of experience by experience."[22] Therefore, to speak of experience is really to listen to experience. To listen to another is to participate in the truth of what she says. Understanding is a participation, "a participation in the stream of tradition, in a moment which mixes past and present."[23] The moment of participation joins the individual to his neighbor as he speaks with integrity, and listens in the manner of one who is oriented to the future, one who would be taught.[24] So understanding is a community of shared meaning sustained by integrity, enabling dialogue. Through dialogue, we re-turn more deeply to our experience in anticipation of our future.

Logos teaches us to speak, to listen. Logos is our teacher. When we open ourselves to logos, our attitude is unlike that of the researcher whose parameters for meaningfulness are control and replication. Our openness to logos is a dialectic of questioning and being put in question, speaking and listening. To dialogue is to listen to, and to speak with our teacher, as our teacher is presented to us in the sound and silence of strangers and friends, work and re-creation, wind and waves.

CHAPTER 5

THE QUESTION OF THEORIZING

But where danger is, grows
The saving power also.

—Hölderlin

We search *for* the meaning of theorizing by searching *through* the meaning of theorizing. We pause before the word as before a monument. Yet, the word abides, not as a relic but as a possibility for us from ancient Greek times. What persists in the word is our quest for what is good in life. We not only speak about theorizing: we theorize. We become the horizon of the word. Blum puts into question the nature and purpose of theorizing:

> Is there any difference between theorizing in order to produce a collective, that is, to justify theory because it leads to the production of a collective, and theorizing as the search for the collective that it presupposes (that makes possible theorizing itself)?[1]

Theory Building

The theorist who sets out "to produce a collective" has a vision of the common good as the agreement which uniformity manifests. Therefore, the theorist is loyal to the standards established by the existing collective as the resource for the research question and method. A central research concern is "How can agreement be achieved in a

problematic situation (a situation of difference)?" A problem
is reconcilable through method, the construction of an "ideal
type" of an actor, that is, the theorist's re-presentation of his
or her rational response in the problematic situation. Through
the creation of an "ideal type" of an actor, the theorist
"assimilates what is good to words."[2] What is good is a
program for action which converts members of the collective
into actors who approximate the ideal type in the problematic
situation. Through their action, the theorist's speech is
converted into an "object of common experience,"[3] as each new
situation is reduced to a variation of the same situation. The
theorist's work is valued according to the efficiency of the
uniform action it sponsors in the problematic situation.

Theory Finding

"Theorizing as the search for the collective that it
presupposes" searches for the good as the agreement which
unity manifests. The good is that which speaks in every
utterance, every gesture (even by absence) but cannot itself
be spoken. The good is therefore the reference for speaking.
The theorist unites the members of the collective in the quest
for their "deep unity,"[4] the concerted questioning of what is
agreed upon but unthought, what is secure in its everyday-
ness. The theorist's central question is not, "How can we
achieve sameness in a situation that highlights difference?"
but, "How can we re-cognize difference in a situation that
is taken for granted?" The theorist is committed to his
difference from each person as the purpose for speaking, the
need for dialogue. The theorist's method, therefore, is not to
reconcile difference through an ideal type of an actor but to
evoke the uniqueness of each individual's experience in a
situation held in common. The task of the theorist is to
transform anecdotes into examples which are "personifica-
tions of the occasion of thinking."[5] Only in a situation that
is critical for the theorist can such examples "come to light."[6]

The deep unity of community is evoked in the sharing
of such examples of experience which are not mine but could

be mine, the understanding: "Yes, life is like that; I, too, have lived." However, theorizing does not end in reverie. Theorizing renews itself in thoughtful action, the commitment: "I, too, will live."

Parsons' Theorizing: Professional Health Care

For nearly five decades, human science researchers have seen the experience of illness through the theory of Talcott Parsons, who used illness as an example for the functional analysis of social systems. According to Parsons,[7] care of the ill is a social role relationship aimed at returning a dysfunctional individual to a functioning state. The patient is, in a sense, a socially deviant individual, unable to fulfill his or her customary role in society because of illness. The doctor is the professional whose technical qualifications grant him the power to return the patient to a functional state. Therefore, the presence of an individual in a doctor's office or emergency ward signifies the inability of the individual to help himself. The individual who chooses in this way to be a patient grants parental-like authority to the doctor to legitimate the suspicion of illness and to prescribe diagnostic and treatment procedures. The patient's being like a child derives not only from the doctor's technical power to cure but also from the physical and emotional onslaught of illness— the patient wants to be cared for.

The patient assumes a socially and emotionally dependent role. The doctor, however, maintains a professional attitude which is characterized by three attributes. *Affective neutrality* is the requirement that the doctor distance himself from the patient; the doctor may sympathize with the patient but does not emphathize with him. *Universalism* is the requirement that the doctor treat all patients equally regardless of available nonmedical information. *Functional specificity* is the requirement that the doctor's sphere of influence be bounded by strictly medical concerns as contrasted with spiritual, financial, or political concerns which are the arena of other social agencies. Thus, Parsons' model of the ideal type of doctor-patient relationship entails a basic mutuality, a meshing of expectations. The doctor is trained and expected to act; the patient acknowledges the doctor's expertise and obeys the doctor's orders.

Critiques of Parsons' Theory

The degree of patient involvement is often greater or less than Parsons' ideal type, according to Szaz and Hollender,[8] who identify three types of patient involvement based on behavioral implications of organic symptoms. The norm identified by Parsons is termed *guidance-cooperation*: the doctor guides, the patient cooperates. Less patient involvement is typified as *activity-passivity*: the doctor acts upon the patient's passive body. Szaz and Hollender compare the relationship between doctor and patient to that between parent and infant. Greater patient involvement is typified as *mutual participation*: the doctor and patient share responsibility. Szaz and Hollender compare the relationship to that between adults where one adult has specialized information that the other needs.

Whereas Parsons and Szaz and Hollender rely on a functional theory of doctor-patient relationships, Freidson[9] theorizes that the structure of interpersonal networks that operates in everyday life is the most important variable in the experience of illness. The patient, a member of the lay health system, consults with relatives, persons with similar complaints, the drug store clerk, books, for example; as well as with the doctor, the representative of the professional health system. Any of these consultants can be a source of diagnosis, treatment, and referrals.

Freidson critiques Parsons for seeing the doctor-patient relationship from the doctor's perspective only and for limiting the analysis of the experience of illness to functional expectations only, thus artificially minimizing the possibility of conflict. The doctor "expects patients to accept what he recommends on his terms; patients seek services on their own terms. In that each seek to gain their own terms, there is conflict."[10]

Within the same frame of reference, Freidson critiques the typology of Szaz and Hollender because it represents a continuum of patient involvement without identifying a similar continuum of doctor involvement. Freidson suggests two other types of doctor-patient relationships which are a logical extension of the continuum: *patient guides—doctor cooperates; patient is active—doctor is passive*. He contends that these two types should not be ignored just because doctors generally reject the possibility of their appropriateness.

Freidson's shift from the analysis of mutual expectations to the analysis of conflicting social systems pivots on the critique of expertise:

> Neither expertise nor the expert who practises it has been examined carefully enough to allow intelligent and self-conscious formulation of the proper role of the expert in free society. Indeed...expertise is more and more in danger of being used as a mask of privilege and power rather than, as it claims, as a mode of advancing public interest.[11]

Joining in this shift are Berger and Luckman, who describe the institution of medicine as "a sub-universe of meaning" that is, a closed system. An "entire legitimating machinery is at work so that laymen will remain laymen, and doctors doctors, and (if at all possible) that both will do so happily."[12] Illich provides similar commentary:

> Neither high income nor long training nor delicate tasks nor social standing is the mark of the professional, but it is his power to determine what shall be needed by his client. The physician, for instance, became a doctor when he left commerce in medicine to the pharmacist and kept prescription for himself.[13]

The discussion of social conflict and legitimating processes loses sight of the person who is a doctor and the person who is a patient. Faceless laypersons confront faceless experts.

Two Revolutionary Experiments

Cousins shows the face of the experience of illness in his book, *Anatomy of an Illness,* which describes his convalescence from a crippling disease.[14] In 1964, an expert diagnosed the disease as progressive paralysis. Cousins decided to fight the unbeatable disease by involving himself in research and treatment. His doctor cooperated with his suggestions for treatment because alternatives provided by medical science were also unproven and because he was a close friend of Cousins' family. Cousins believed that negative emotions have detrimental effects on health so he planned to cultivate the positive emotions. First, though, he discontinued using pain killers which left toxic wastes in his body producing side effects such as hives, and reduced his body's ability to fight the disease. When the pain became intense, he watched Candid Camera and Marx Brothers movies. The laughter produced an anaesthetic effect and he was able to sleep for as long as two hours. In 1974, Cousins met the expert who told him he had progressive paralysis. The expert was anxious to know about Cousins' remarkable recovery.

> It all began, I said, when I decided that some experts don't really know enough to make a pronouncement of doom on a human being. And I said I hoped they would be careful about what they said to others; they might be believed and that could be the beginning of the end.[15]

Doctor Robert Mendelsohn, chairman of the Medical Licensing Committee for Illinois and associate professor of preventative medicine and community health in the School of Medicine, University of Illinois, advocates "new medicine,"[16] an ethical system made viable through family and community. Doctor Mendelsohn theorizes that the "determinants of health" are "life, love, and courage."[17] Supported by the love of family and community, the individual finds courage to be responsible for one's own health. The "new doctor" is a "lifeguard" who "acknowledges nature as the prime healer."[18] The new medical school will have Departments of Ethics and

Justice as well as a Department of Iatrogenic Disease. The dominant ethic in the education and practise of the doctor is regard for the rights and dignity of each human being.

Where Does "Theorizing in Order to Produce a Collective" Lead?

Parsons' theory collects doctors and patients in a functional relationship. Inasmuch as a functional relationship is not sufficient for the everyday life of illness, Parsons' theory turns us to the logos of the experience of illness. Because of the turning, Heidegger sees in the "danger" of technology, that is, function as the only criterion for relationship, the possibility for the "saving power."[19]

Turning from the experience of medical care guided by Parsons' theory, Cousins and Doctor Mendelsohn seek the logos of the experience of illness in responsibility—responsibility for oneself and for the other. Cousins finds that assuming responsibility for his own health care with the support of his family and family doctor activates the body's healing mechanisms. His responsibility is tied to his attitude to learn all he can about his illness and possible remedies, and to obey biological and emotional laws governing health. Doctor Mendelsohn advocates that professional medical care be a support system that pivots around the health needs of the family. The responsibility of family members for each other's health includes such essential concerns as nutrition and dedicating time for family activities; in short, putting family first.

This fundamental responsibility of the individual in community reminds us of the dedication of Heraclitus to logos. More recently, Levinas has theorized that responsibility is a *prima facie* accountability for the well-being of one's neighbor. In the look, one becomes interchangeable with anyone, yet because one is unique, this interchangeability is not like another but for another. This responsibility for another is not bound to personal interest or any pre-established system. It is a subjection to the good which shows itself in "the unforeseeable response of the chosen one."[20]

Who is the chosen one? And what is the nature of one's calling? Is the medical doctor truly an expert with the power to cure or a "lifeguard" who "acknowledges nature as the prime healer?" Is the patient dependent on the doctor or responsible for one's own care? Is the family during illness an emotional backwater or the fulcrum of existence? Are these theories mutually exclusive? In many ways, modern medical care images Parsons' theory. How can we image what belongs to logos, the difference that matters?

Heidegger's Theorizing: The Homecoming Journey

The theorist's journey has been an allegory for the search for logos, the difference that matters, since ancient Greek times. "Probably the earliest use of the word theoros strongly evoked the components of theo and eros," Jager writes, "to read approximately 'he who regards and observes (the will of) God.'"[21]

Where shall we go to regard and observe the will of God? Shall we journey to Mount Olympus to view the temple ruins? And what message shall we bring back? Is there anything left to say? POLAROID shows us the value of temple ruins. Just as an INSTAMATIC photograph of temple ruins is framed by many tourists as a resource for 'travel talk' without a perspective concerning the temple, so we are "enframed"[22] in a narrow perspective on life: we take for granted that anything is a resource only; we do not think to question the essence of the thing.

A journey requires a home base—a place of departure, a place to return to. The ancient Greek theorist knew the soil of that place, his home, his dwelling place. We have no place for rootedness, for learning to know the soil of our existence. The temple ruins are as close as an enframed photograph but family and friends are distant. Jager writes, "Meaning grows out of loyalty to origins. All journeying and every detail of an itinerary must refer to the sphere of dwelling. A journey cut off from its source degenerates into eternal departure."[23]

Heidegger calls the journey that is eternal departure, *verfall*,[24] a falling away from our self. Such a journey is marked by "collective indiscrimination" and inauthentic speech. "Everyone is the other and no one is himself. . . . The being that is us is eroded into commonality; it subsides to a 'oneness' within and among a collective public, herd-like 'theyness.' "[25] Responsibility is relegated to 'them.' Everyone is guided by the values of 'them.' We live in fear of what 'they' prescribe for us. We search for novelty to make life worthwhile. We have become resource-ful overseers of the human resource.

Marcel describes the same situation as a "devitalization process" where the collectivization of individuals results in the "reduction of a personality to an official identity. . . What is going to become of this inner life?" he asks. "What does a creature who is thus pushed about from pillar to post, ticketed, docketed, labelled, become for himself and in himself?"[26] And how does an "official identity" speak? When speech has lost its relationship with the essence of what is spoken about, speech deteriorates to noise, idle talk, ambiguity.

Yet, verfall is an essential part of being in the world, according to Heidegger: being in the world necessitates being with others. Verfall, which is not a genuine being with others (because we are not genuine) generates a deep longing for something more. Experiencing what is inauthentic, we dare to hope for what is authentic. Steiner, who interprets Heidegger's writing, articulates our thoughts:

> Desire and hope are the reaching-forward of care. Thus care underlies and necessitates 'the possibility of being free' [authentic]. The careless man and the uncaring are not free. It is care that makes human existence meaningful, that makes a man's life signify.[27]

CHAPTER 6

A PATHWAY FOR THEORIZING

There is a way of thinking,
in contact with the event,
which seeks its concrete structure.

—Merleau-Ponty

Wonder at What Is: Language and Truthfulness

We observe the difference between a diamond stone and a glass stone that are identically cut and mounted. The diamond is truly a diamond, the glass is truly not a diamond, though it may appear so. Each stone has the possibility of a genuine appraisal (its own) and the possibility of a false appraisal (if one is taken for the other). When the stone is, in fact, a diamond, and we say, "This stone is a diamond," we have expressed a true proposition. The truth (correctness) of the proposition is found in the truth (correctness) of the matter. The proposition presents the matter, the proposition lets "the thing stand opposed as object."[1] But, asks Heidegger, what is the meaning of 'let' whereby the proposition "subordinates itself to the directive that it speaks of beings such as they are"?[2]

'Let' provides an opening for the shining of the essence of the diamond: the proposition, 'This stone is a diamond' lets be "what something is, as it is."[3] 'Let' is the ground of the possibility of correctness. 'Let' is the freedom of the object to be what it is. "The essence of truth is freedom."[4]

The Greek word for the shimmering freedom of the essence of an object is *aletheia*, usually translated 'truth,' although more literally, "unconcealment."[5] "Unconcealment"

83

helps us think beyond truth as correctness to the ground of correctness, freedom, an enabling of unconcealment. We are the place where all beings are unconcealed. We are possessed by the freedom of the object to disclose itself. Therefore, our manner towards all beings is openness: we live in the question. History ever begins with the question.

Our manner of being among beings is openness. The manner of being of all other beings is unconcealment. Why, then, has our relationship to beings through history not become fixed in absolute knowledge? To consider this question, we must search the other side of openness and the other side of unconcealment: Heidegger names the other side of openness, "errancy"; the other side of unconcealment, "concealment."⁶ 'Errancy' is our predisposition to satisfy our wants and needs as easily as possible, to ask superficial questions because everything is already familiar. Errancy closes us off from the unconcealing of beings: when we are a closed place, the essence of beings is sheltered in conceal-ment. We are always the place of an opening-closing so that the unconcealing of beings is always sheltered in concealing. Therefore, the mystery of being is preserved from us and for us.

Heidegger proposes that "the essence of truth is the truth of essence."⁷ "The essence of truth" means "accordance between knowledge and beings" (correctness). "The truth of essence" means "sheltering that lightens" (*aletheia*). 'Is' means "lets essentially unfold" (freedom). The origin of wonder at what is, is freedom, the questioning openness of letting-be what is disclosing itself.

Just as a life of openness to the object cannot be demanded, so a life of openness to the other cannot be demanded. "How could a life of dialogue be demanded?" Buber writes. "There is no ordering of dialogue. It is not that you are to answer but that you are able."⁸ How can we respond to the appeal, 'You are able?' How can we be an open place?

Speech in the Light of Logos:
The Work of Art and Theorizing

The artist is an open place for the unconcealing-concealing of being. Truth happens in the work of art, the artist's place, the place where unconcealing and concealing strive.[9] Heidegger gives us a description of Van Gogh's painting of peasant shoes. The shoes stand nowhere, anywhere, yet never on the canvas. The canvas disappears, not under the paint, but with the paint, with the artist, concealed in the unconcealing of the shoes. For, in the work of art, the shoes re-present the world of the peasant woman.

> From the dark opening of the worn insides of the shoes the toilsome tread of the worker stares forth. In the stiffly rugged heaviness of the shoes there is the accumulated tenacity of her slow trudge through the far-spreading and ever-uniform furrows of the field swept by a raw wind. In the leather lie the dampness and richness of the soil. Under the shoes slides the loneliness of the fieldpath as evening falls. In the shoes vibrates the silent call of the earth. . .[10]

In the work of art, the shoes that the peasant woman wears without thinking about it bring forth a world that we recognize, a world we assumed we did not know. How does the truth of the peasant woman's world come into play in Van Gogh's painting and in Heidegger's theorizing?

The phrase, 'come into play,' signifies that play is a clue to the origin of the work of art. Play detaches us from everything, then gives us back the whole of our being.[11] For example, the world of play envelops the child who plays house: the child disappears into an adult identity. The inner consistency of the world of play constrains everyone who enters to obey the rules of play. Willing parents 'visit' the child for a cup of tea. The play takes place for the child as well as in the child. To say that the child is pretending to be an adult misses the significance of the child's re-presentation of what it means to the child to be an adult. Parents recognize themselves in the child's play and return to the everyday world a bit wiser for the experience.

"Human play finds its true perfection in being art," writes Gadamer.[12] Just as the playing child is set apart in a closed world—a world with its own compelling structure—so the work of art is a closed world. The two complementary aspects of the structure of this closed world found the permanence of the work of art in its temporality: the work of art is a meaningful whole which can be repeatedly re-presented; only in each re-presentation of the work of art can the meaningful whole be unconcealed. Like a tree through the seasons and the years, the work of art retains its identity in the changing aspects of itself. "It has its being only in becoming and return."[13]

The artist is the open place for the becoming of the work of art. But, like the playing child, the artist disappears in the play of the work of art. Unlike the playing child, this disappearance is not just for himself but for everyone. The disappearance of the artist for everyone is the perfection of play: it enables us to be the open place for the return of the play of the work of art.

However, the theorist fulfills the purpose of the work of art by being there thoughtfully on our behalf. "Theoria is a true sharing," Gadamer writes, "being totally involved in and carried away by what one sees."[14] Participation in the world of the work of art estranges the theorist from the taken-for-grantedness of the everyday world. "What existed previously no longer exists," Gadamer writes. "But also that what now exists, what represents itself in the play of art is what is lasting and true."[15] For example, Van Gogh's painting of peasant shoes fills us with the spirit of the peasant woman's world. Heidegger's theorizing analyzes his experience of seeing the peasant shoes as for the first time in the work of art; severed from their common ground, the peasant shoes are grounded in their essence, their equipmental reliability.[16] The theorist leaves home (what is familiar and taken-for-granted) to come home (to what is familiar and appreciated). Like the child whose play at being an adult 'speaks' to the parents, the play of the work of art 'speaks' to the theorist. The "joy of recognition," Gadamer writes, is that "more becomes known that is already known. In recognition what we know emerges, as if through an illumination."[17]

The artist re-searches the temporal for what is "lasting and true" in a way that transforms what is lasting and true "into an image or a form."[18] For example, we see Michelangelo's Pièta, we hear Bach's chorales, and we read Milton's poetry. The theorist returns to the community to speak the life of one who lives the truth of the subject matter. This translation of the personal experience of the work of art into the life we can share is expressed through the theme. The dwelling place of thematic research is the question, "What belongs to logos, to our community, to each other?"

Kierkegaard's Theorizing: The Freedom of Faith

In *Fear and Trembling*,[19] a phenomenology of faith, Kierkegaard journeys to the estranged ground of the Biblical account of the faith of Abraham. "Finally, he forgot everything else because of it; his soul had but one wish, to see Abraham, but one longing, to have witnessed that event."[20] "Occupied" by the "shudder of an idea,"[21] Kierkegaard becomes the open place of a question: Who can understand Abraham?

> And God did tempt [test] Abraham, and said unto him, Abraham: and he said, Behold, here I am. And he said, Take now thy son, thine only son Isaac, whom thou lovest, and get thee into the land of Moriah; and offer him there for a burnt offering upon one of the mountains which I will tell thee of.
>
> And Abraham rose up early in the morning, and saddled his ass, and took two of his young men with him, and Isaac his son, and clave the wood for the burnt offering, and rose up, and went unto the place of which God had told him.
>
> Then on the third day Abraham lifted up his eyes, and saw the place afar off. . .
>
> And Isaac spake unto Abraham his father, and said, My father: and he said, Here am I, my son. And he said, Behold the fire and the wood: but where is the lamb for a burnt offering?
>
> And Abraham said, My son, God will provide himself a lamb for a burnt offering: so they went both of them together.

And they came to the place which God had told him of; and Abraham built an altar there, and laid the wood in order, and bound Isaac his son, and laid him on the altar upon the wood.

And Abraham stretched forth his hand, and took the knife to slay his son.

And the angel of the Lord called unto him out of heaven, and said, Abraham, Abraham: and he said, Here am I. And he said, Lay not thine hand upon the lad, neither do thou any thing unto him: for now I know that thou fearest God, seeing thou hast not withheld thy son, thine only son, from me.

And Abraham lifted up his eyes, and looked, and beheld behind him a ram caught in a thicket by his horns, and Abraham went and took the ram, and offered him up for a burnt offering in the stead of his son.[22]

Theorizing with Examples

Kierkegaard strives to show how Abraham could have lived this experience with Isaac, with a story of how a mother could live the experience of weaning with her child.[23] In love, the mother withholds her warmth and sustenance from the child at the right time. And the child lives on by faith in the mother, for who else is the source of sustenance?

Abraham lived by faith, sojourning in a foreign land, daily bereft of the companionship and language of his kinfolk. His homeland was the promise of God. Abraham grew old waiting for the fulfillment of the promise, the birth of his only son, Isaac, through whom his descendants would be named inheritors of the promised land. And each time Abraham looked on Isaac his son, he saw God his father. How could Abraham ever be weaned from one without losing all?

Theorizing with Thematic Questions

Love transforms Abraham's ordeal from murder into tragedy; faith transforms it from tragedy into a "holy and God-pleasing act, a paradox that gives Isaac back to Abraham again."[24] Kierkegaard researches three themes of faith that come to light in his response to the Biblical text.

1. "Is There a Teleological Suspension of the Ethical?"[25] "In ethical terms, Abraham's relation to Isaac is quite simply this: the father shall love the son more than himself."[26] If Abraham had sacrificed himself, all human beings would understand the selfless act, for he was the father of Isaac—he loved his son more than himself. If Abraham had turned back at any time during the ordeal, all human beings would understand the rational act, for he was the father of Isaac—he loved the son whom he had seen more than God whom he had not seen. More deeply, how could Abraham love Isaac less by loving God more? Yet who can understand Abraham? He was the father of faith—he was willing to lose all, and, at every moment, he believed he would receive all back again.

2. "Is There an Absolute Duty to God?"[27] The hero relinquishes one for the sake of all. Abraham relinquishes all for the sake of One. "For God's sake and—the two are wholly identical—for his own sake. He does it for God's sake because God demands this proof of his faith; he does it for his own sake so that he can prove it."[28] The hero's relationship to the absolute is determined by his relationship to the ethical, his duty to man. Abraham's relationship to the ethical is determined by his relationship to the absolute, his duty to God. "The paradox of faith, then, is this," Kierkegaard writes, "that the single individual is higher than the universal."[29]

3. "Was it Ethically Defensible for Abraham to Conceal His Understanding from Sarah, Eliezer, and from Isaac?"[30] The hero speaks a universal language. Abraham speaks "in tongues."[31] He speaks the truth that conceals the truth from Isaac, his son. He keeps silence with Sarah, his wife, and Eliezer, his servant. Kierkegaard writes that he longed to "go along on the three-day journey when Abraham rode with sorrow before him and Isaac beside him."[32] For he recognized the sorrow of silence—the sorrow of the individual without community. Abraham is cut off from all for the sake of the One who justifies him. Yet, at every moment, faith transforms the ordeal into personal victory. Who can understand Abraham?

Responding to Kierkegaard's Theorizing

The question, "Who can understand Abraham?" is permeated by the question, "How ought we to live?" This question is given to us as a possibility for living in faith. There is nothing in the world that we can see or touch that has the name, faith. When we speak of faith, we name a manner of openness, a way of living in the question. We name a man, Abraham. Research in the human sciences begins with the name of a human being, the recollection of a life. This life is, in some sense, not only one life but our life; it is our ordeal, our possibility.

Abraham is ("lets essentially unfold") the open place for the unconcealing of the beginning: faith. Faith is free to be what it is in Abraham's life of obedience to God. Kierkegaard, a human being like Abraham, is put into question by the themes of faith that 'speak' through his theorizing as he dialogues with these themes. For example, in response to his third thematic question, Kierkegaard omits the Bible verse in which Abraham speaks plainly of his faith (but not of his ordeal) to his young men: ". . . Abide ye here with the ass; and I and the lad will go yonder and worship, and come again to you."[33] So Kierkegaard's writing is not the last word but an other word. Forever, Abraham begins his homecoming journey in the lives of all who want to read with understanding.

Taking Up the Journey

We ask, "Can we understand the life of illness?" More deeply, we wonder, "How ought we to live?" And more incessantly, we ponder, "Why illness?" We have journeyed thus far in an effort to learn how to articulate these questions of the heart. Our pathway intersected and paralleled the paths of many who have gone before. The creative work of laying down this path responds to their creative work. For example, Heraclitus opened the possibilities of the dialectic, "All is one," for us. Gadamer kept the possibilities open by showing us that pain enables us to live in these questions. Blum's research through theorizing led us to the pathway described by Heidegger as the homecoming journey. With Kierkegaard's help, we witnessed the homecoming journey in the Biblical account of the life of Abraham. And with van Manen's help, we take up the journey as research for living.[34] We want to understand the homecoming journey by means of illness in the lives of family, friends, and medical professionals by reading and sharing literary works of art.

Together, we will read excerpts from literature describing the experience of illness. The subject matter of each excerpt shines through its situatedness in a historical context and 'speaks' into our context in a way that transcends our context, too. At the same time, the concealing-revealing of the subject matter binds the unknown author to us in a context of giving. "The sharing of meaning with integrity is the generous gift of the creative writer," writes Hunsberger. "Our own experience is reconfirmed and clarified, as well as extended."[35] In response, we too, are willing to "share meaning with integrity." Life speaks to life and we respond, not with a "bald re-enactment," but with Hoy's "new creation of understanding."[36]

CHAPTER 7

IVAN ILYITCH: ONE AGAINST THE OTHER SEARCHES FOR THE OTHER

The true office of any faith
is to give life a meaning
that death cannot destroy.

—Leo Tolstoy

On *The Death of Ivan Ilyitch*: The Chaplain Speaks

In *The Death of Ivan Ilyitch*,[1] Leo Tolstoy portrays Ivan as a husband, father, friend, judge, master, Catholic, and poker enthusiast. All of Ivan's pursuits are cast in shadow by the events of his death, a death made lonely by the pride of his life, propriety, which sets him against the other even as he desperately searches for the other.

Encounter with Death

i. *Knowing without believing.*
ii. *What does mortal mean to one who is not suffering death?*
iii. *Ivan reflects on his life because of his illness.*
iv. *Life is understood in the fullness of particular experiences.*
v. *Feelings and ideas are personal possessions. Why "ought" Ivan die?*

i. At the bottom of his heart Ivan Ilyitch knew that he was dying; but so far from growing used to this idea, he simply did not grasp it—he was utterly unable to grasp it.

ii. The example of the syllogism that he had learned in Kiseveter's logic—Caius is a man, men are mortal, therefore

93

Caius is mortal—had seemed to him all his life correct only as regards Caius, but not at all as regards himself. In that case it was a question of Caius, a man, an abstract man, and it was perfectly true, but he was not Caius, and was not an abstract man; he had always been a creature quite, quite different from all others;

iii, iv. He had been little Vanya with a mamma and papa, and Mitya and Volodya, with playthings and a coachman and a nurse; afterwards with Katenka, with all the joys and griefs and ecstasies of childhood, boyhood, and youth. What did Caius know of the smell of the leathern ball Vanya had been so fond of? Had Caius kissed his mother's hand like that? Caius had not heard the silk rustle of his mother's skirts. He had not made a riot at school over the pudding. Had Caius been in love like that? Could Caius preside over the sittings of the court?

v. And Caius certainly was mortal, and it was right for him to die; but for me, little Vanya, Ivan Ilyitch, with all my feelings and ideas—for me it's a different matter. And it cannot be that I ought to die. That would be too awful. (pp. 43, 44)

To whom can we appeal concerning Ivan's life, moments treasured like polished stones, hidden in a box—"the smell of the leathern ball," "the silk rustle of his mother's skirts," "a riot at school over the pudding?" Are these not treasures worth defending? Yet death treats Ivan's life as a common thing: death laughs at Ivan and his jewels. The sentence of death cannot be appealed. Ivan, like Caius, must die. Ivan knows his death is imminent but he cannot believe it. He cannot relinquish his jewels, his very own jewels, his very own Vanya.

Against Death

i.   *The fear of 'It'*;
ii. *Hiding from 'It'*;
iii. *Compelled by 'It'*;
iv. *Diversions from 'It'*;
v.   *Failure.*

i. It came and stood confronting him and looked at him, and he felt turned to stone, and the light died away in his eyes, and he began to ask himself again, 'Can it be that It is the only truth?' And his colleagues and his subordinates saw with surprise and distress that he, the brilliant, subtle judge, was losing the thread of his speech, was making blunders.

ii. He shook himself, tried to regain his self control, and got somehow to the end of the sitting, and went home with the painful sense that his judicial labours could not as of old hide from him what he wanted to hide; that he could not by means of his official work escape from It.

iii. And the worst of it was that It drew him to itself not for him to do anything in particular, but simply for him to look at It straight in the face, to look at It and, doing nothing, suffer unspeakably.

iv. And to save himself from this, Ivan Ilyitch sought amusements, other screens, and these screens he found, and for a little while they did seem to save him;

v. but soon again they were not so much broken down as let the light through, as though It pierced through everything, and there was nothing that could shut It off. (p. 45)

When is death present? When is it absent? 'It' is always present. Our screen of activities and amusements cannot veil 'It.' "At the origin of diversion, of the will to be diverted or amused at any price, there is an attempt to escape, but from what? It can only be from oneself," writes Marcel.[2] This hide-and-seek is played like the children's game: when 'It' catches us in our hiding place, we become 'It.' "Ultimately, we cannot keep up the deception," says the chaplain.[3] Death wears our own face.

Against Deception

i. *Try persuasion*;
ii. *Try denial*;
iii. *Try routinizing illness*;
iv. *The need for honesty.*

i. Ivan Ilyitch's great misery was due to the deception that
for some reason or other every one kept up with him—that
he was simply ill, and not dying, and that he need only keep
quiet and follow the doctor's orders, and then some great
change for the better would be the result. He knew that
whatever they might do, there would be no result except
more agonizing sufferings and death. And he was made
miserable by this lie, made miserable at their refusing to
acknowledge what they all knew and he knew, by persisting
in lying over him about his awful position, and in forcing
him too to take part in this lie.

ii. Lying, lying, this lying carried on over him on the eve
of his death, and destined to bring that terrible, solemn act
of his death down to the level of all their visits, curtains
[Ivan was injured hanging curtains], sturgeons for dinner
[doctor's orders]. . .was a horrible agony for Ivan Ilyitch.

iii. And, strange to say, many times when they had been
going through the regular performance over him, he had
been within a hair's breadth of screaming at them: 'Cease
your lying! You know, and I know, that I'm dying; so do,
at least, give over lying!'

iv. But he had never had the spirit to do this. (p. 50)

The experience of dying is reduced to a parody of diet and
rest. Everyone participates in the play. We know our parts
by heart. With all our heart, each of us does not want to die.
With all our heart, the chaplain says, "each of us faces the
terrible fact of death alone."

The Struggle for Truth

i. *Who cares?*
ii. *Who comforts?*
iii. *Who perpetuates the falsity?*

i. Apart from this deception, or in consequence of it, what
made the greatest misery for Ivan Ilyitch was that no one
felt for him as he would have liked them to feel for him.
At certain moments, after prolonged suffering, Ivan Ilyitch,
ashamed as he would have been to own it, longed more than

anything for some one to feel sorry for him, as for a sick child. He longed to be petted, kissed, and wept over, as children are petted and comforted. He knew that he was an important member of the law-courts, that he had a beard turning grey, and that therefore it was impossible. But still he longed for it.

ii. And in his relations with Gerasim there was something approaching to that. And that was why being with Gerasim was a comfort to him. Ivan llyitch longs to weep, longs to be petted and wept over, and then there comes in a colleague, Shebek;

iii. and instead of weeping and being petted, Ivan Ilyitch puts on his serious, severe, earnest face, and from mere inertia gives his views on the effect of the last decision in the Court of Appeal, and obstinately insists upon them. This falsity around him and within him did more than anything to poison Ivan Ilyitch's last days. (p. 51)

This desperate loneliness is overcome when we share our moments with each other. Just holding a hand is "a conversation of common experience," says the chaplain. Yet we continue to engage in the habitual play that we condemn by disengaging our life and death from each other. We retreat from death with proud words and sophisticated manner. And the play goes on.

The Doctor Gives Hope

i. *Medical detail veils the lived-through quality of the struggle against illness.*
ii. *The patient 'listens' to the doctor's manner for a sign of hope.*
iii. *Pity is a response to hope.*

i. At half-past eleven the celebrated doctor came. Again came the sounding, and then grave conversation in his presence and in the other room about the kidney and the appendix, and questions and answers, with such an air of significance, that again, instead of the real question of life and death, which was now the only one that confronted

him, the question that came uppermost was of the kidney
and the appendix, which were doing something not as they
ought to do, and were for that reason being attacked by
Mihail Danilovitch and the celebrated doctor, and forced
to mend their ways.

ii. The celebrated doctor took leave of him with a serious,
but not a hopeless face. And to the timid question that Ivan
Ilyitch addressed to him while he lifted his eyes, shining
with terror and hope, up towards him, Was there a chance
of recovery? He answered that he could not answer for it,
but that there was a chance.

iii. The look of hope with which Ivan Ilyitch watched the
doctor out was so piteous that, seeing it, Praskovya
Fyodorovna positively burst into tears, as she went out of
the door to hand the celebrated doctor his fee in the next
room. (p. 56)

The chaplain observes that "the doctor gives a little hope,
not very much hope," and Ivan's wife gives the doctor the fee.
How much does a little hope cost? How much does a little
hope give? A little hope fills Ivan with gratitude. The presence
of someone who is hopeful provides a moment of companionship on the "terribly perilous, trying journey," says the
chaplain. The doctor cares enough to give a little hope. The
wife cares enough to pay the fee, and she responds to Ivan's
gratitude with tears. For a moment, Ivan is not alone.

Against God
i.   *The tumult of helplessness, loneliness, cruelty,*
ii. *punishment,*
iii. *senselessness,*
iv. *quelled by silence.*

i. he could restrain himself no longer, and cried like a child.
He cried at his own helplessness, at his awful loneliness,
at the cruelty of people, at the cruelty of God, at the absence
of God.

ii. 'Why hast Thou done all this? What brought me to this?
Why, why torture me so horribly?'

iii. He did not expect an answer, and wept indeed that there was and could be no answer. The pain grew more acute again, but he did not stir, did not call. He said to himself, 'Come, more then; come, strike me! But what for? What have I done to Thee? What for?'

iv. Then he was still, ceased weeping, held his breath, and was all attention; he listened, as it were, not to a voice uttering sounds, but the voice of his soul, to the current of thoughts that rose up within him. (p. 60)

The experience of dying gives us the opportunity to be more fully conscious of life. "We pray," says the chaplain, "Spare us from death with our boots on." Yet, at this moment in the experience of dying, Ivan is angry at God. The Latin word for anger, *angere*, means 'to press together, throttle, torment.'[4] Ivan's life is pressed together into this moment of helplessness; he is throttled by the fear of death, and life; he is tormented by his loneliness. Convinced of the absence of God, he seeks the presence of God more earnestly than ever before. Ivan Ilyitch, the fluent judge, stands in the dock. Ivan listens.

Listening to the Voice of Conscience

i.   *Is to suffer not to live?*
ii. *A true response to the voice of conscience.*
iii. *A false response to the voice of conscience.*

i. 'What is it you want?' was the first clear idea able to be put into words that he grasped. 'What? Not to suffer, to live,' he answered.

ii. And again he was plunged into attention so intense that even the pain did not distract him. 'To live? Live how?' the voice of his soul was asking. 'Why, live as I used to live before—happily and pleasantly.'
'As you used to live before—happily and pleasantly?' queried the voice. And he began going over in his imagination the best moments of his pleasant life. But, strange to say, all these best moments of his pleasant life seemed now not at all what they had seemed then. All—except the first

memories of childhood—there, in his childhood there had
been something really pleasant in which one could have
lived if it had come back. But the creature who had this
pleasant experience was no more; it was like a memory of
some one else. (p. 60)

iii. 'But if one could at least comprehend what it's for? Even
that's impossible. It could be explained if one were to say
that I hadn't lived as I ought. But that can't be alleged,'
he said to himself, thinking of all the regularity, correctness, and propriety of his life. 'That really can't be
admitted,' he said to himself, his lips smiling ironically as
though some one could see his smile and be deceived by
it. 'No explanation! Agony, death... What for?' (pp. 63, 64)

Ivan listens and begins to hear the meaning of a happy
and pleasant life. Yet, Ivan's resentment is increased by the
awareness that his propriety (L. *proprietas*, 'property')[5] does
not seem to have any significance now: he resents that his
propriety has left him facing death empty-handed. His proper
marriage, his proper manner in court, his proper artifacts at
home—one breaks as easily as the other. And they all break
at the same time. "We sit like so many spoiled children,"
writes Boulding, "with all our splintered and lifeless utopias
scattered around us like so many broken toys... What is
hurting is that it is the day after Christmas, and we have
lost our sense of the transcendent."[6] "In bewilderment and
anger, Ivan wonders, Does it really matter at all?," the
chaplain says. Yet Ivan clings to his standard: he smiles his
proper smile.

Against Self and Family

i.　*Life is entrusted to each person for good.*
ii.　*Recognition of deception as a way of life.*
iii.　*Physical and spiritual agony intertwine.*

i. 'But if it's so,' he said to himself, 'and I am leaving life
with the consciousness that I have lost all that was given
me, and there's no correcting it, then what?' He lay on his
back and began going over his whole life entirely anew.

When he saw the footman in the morning, then his wife, then his daughter, then the doctor, every movement they made, every word they uttered, confirmed for him the terrible truth that had been revealed to him in the night.

ii. In them he saw himself, saw all in which he had lived, and saw distinctly that it was all not the right thing; it was a horrible, vast deception that concealed both life and death. This consciousness intensified his physical agonies, multiplied them tenfold. He groaned and tossed from side to side and pulled at the covering over him.

iii. It seemed to him that it was stifling him and weighing him down. And for that he hated them. (p. 66)

Ivan is also angry at others. In the morning he sees them, watches them pass by: footman, wife, daughter, doctor. "There is no communication, no reaching out on either side," says the chaplain. Physical discomfort is magnified tenfold because no one cares enough to relieve it. Consequently, Ivan hates them because the covering over him is "stifling him and weighing him down." Propriety is stifling him and weighing him down. "Ivan's anger expresses itself in hatred. Hatred expresses itself in denial," says the chaplain. Ivan forsakes his propriety but he has nothing else to replace it. He has no other footman, or wife, or daughter, or doctor. Ivan is alone.

The Minister Gives Hope

i. *Doubt causes suffering, the light of hope opens up the future.*
ii. *Life is precious again.*

i. When the priest came and confessed him he was softened, felt as if it were a relief from his doubts, and consequently from his sufferings, and there came a moment of hope. He began once more thinking of the intestinal appendix and the possibility of curing it. He took the sacrament with tears in his eyes. When they laid him down again after the sacrament for a minute, he felt comfortable, and again the hope of life sprang up. He began to think about the operation which had been suggested to him.

ii. 'To live, I want to live,' he said to himself. (p. 67)

Into Ivan's life comes a person who is a symbol of "acceptance as the release from resentment, peace as the release from anger," says the chaplain. The priest is an intermediary between God and man. "He gives the opportunity to ask for forgiveness," the chaplain continues. The sense of reassurance in his presence gives Ivan new courage. The anger that had destroyed hope is dissipated: hope is rekindled. The light in his parents' eyes for a little boy who wanted forgiveness is true for him yet. "To live, I want to live." This time, Ivan will be Vanya.

From Hope to Hopelessness

i.   *Non-involvement;*
ii. *defeat.*
iii. *When hope leaves, fear and doubt become terrorists.*
iv. *Hopelessness.*

i. His wife came in to congratulate him; she uttered the customary words and added—

'It's quite true, isn't it, that you're better?'

Without looking at her, he said, 'Yes.'

ii. The expression of his face as he uttered that 'Yes' was terrible. After uttering that 'Yes,' looking her straight in the face, he turned on to his face, with a rapidity extraordinary in his weakness, and shrieked

'Go away, go away, let me be!'

iii. From that moment there began the scream that never ceased for three days, and was so awful that through two closed doors one could not hear it without horror. At the moment when he answered his wife he grasped that he had fallen, that there was no return, that the end had come, quite the end, while doubt was still as unsolved, still remained doubt.

iv. 'Oo! Oo-o! Oo!' he screamed in varying intonations. He had begun screaming, 'I don't want to!' and so had gone on screaming in the same vowel sound—oo! (pp. 67, 68)

Ivan's wife has "no ability or desire to support him," says the chaplain. She fills the silence with empty words. In the presence of each other, Ivan and his wife are each alone. "The peace and hope that had just been received sacramentally through one who symbolized the Sacrament of Life, seems to be snuffed out so easily," the chaplain says. He shares the experience of a friend, dying of brain cancer, who asked for "all the help I can get, not just one moment." His hope was nourished daily by loving family and friends. He died hopefully. "The more daring the hope, the more imaginative the hope, the more we can face the future," says the chaplain. There is no daring hope for Ivan. He is a man without community. Even the sound of his last cries are shut out. There are two doors that bar the way: one is Ivan, the other is his family and friends.

The Miracle of Forgiveness

i.   *Experiencing forgiveness*:
ii. *forgetting self,*
iii. *expressing forgiveness.*

> i. At that very moment Ivan Ilyitch had rolled into the hole, and caught sight of the light, and it was revealed to him that his life had not been what it ought to have been, but that could still be set right. He asked himself, 'What is the right thing?'—and became quiet, listening. Then he felt someone was kissing his hand. He opened his eyes and glanced at his son. He felt sorry for him. His wife went up to him. He glanced at her. She was gazing at him with open mouth, the tears unwiped streaming over her nose and cheeks, a look of despair on her face. He felt sorry for her.

> ii. 'Yes, I'm making them miserable,' he thought. 'They're sorry, but it will be better for them when I die.' He would have said this, but had not the strength to utter it. 'Besides, why speak, I must act,' he thought. With a glance to his wife he pointed to his son and said

> iii. 'Take away... sorry for him ...And you too. ...' He tried to say 'forgive,' but said 'forgo'...and too weak to correct himself, shook his hand, knowing that He would understand whose understanding mattered. (p. 69)

The chaplain recalls that Bunyan wrote, "One seeks the light over the wicket gate." Ivan asks, "What is the right thing?" and enters the gate. He listens for the voice of God; he ceases to pity himself. "Ivan comes through resentment, anger, hate, denial: the touch of hope, received in the Sacrament, rekindles faith," says the chaplain. And faith asks forgiveness. Ivan expresses sorrow for those he once denied. Through his difficult journey, Ivan has gotten free of his propriety. He has found that hope is a relationship "between him who gives and him who receives. This exchange is the mark of all spiritual life," writes Marcel.[7] Vanya lives.

Set Free

i.   *To set them free.*
ii. *Set free from the fear of pain,*
iii. *set free from the fear of death.*
iv. *Set free for joy.*

> i. And all at once it became clear to him that what had tortured him and would not leave him was suddenly dropping away all at once on both sides and on ten sides and on all sides. He was sorry for them, must act so that they might not suffer. Set them free and be free himself of those agonies. 'How right and how simple!' he thought. 'And the pain?' he asked himself. 'Where's it gone? Eh, where are you, pain?'
>
> He began to watch for it.
>
> ii. 'Yes, here it is. Well what of it, let the pain be.'
>
> iii. 'And death. Where is it?' He looked for his old accustomed terror of death, and did not find it. 'Where is it? What death?' There was no terror, because death was not either. In the place of death there was light. 'So this is it!' he suddenly exclaimed aloud.
>
> iv. 'What joy!' (p. 69)

The question, 'What is the right thing?' has become a hopeful quest. As Ivan is swallowed in light, he realizes that there is more to his wife and son than propriety because he has found more than propriety in himself. He has found faith. On his death-bed, Ivan wants to "set them free." And suddenly, the pain and death that had harrassed him become companions of light: pain reminds him he is still on this earth; death reminds him he is not long for this earth.

The Meaning of the Last Moment

i. *The meaning of forgiveness does not suffer change.*
ii. *Life is over.*
iii. *What is over?*
iv. *Ivan has already died to falsity, propriety, hatred, doubt.*

> i. To him all this passed in a single instant, and the meaning of that instant suffered no change after. For those present his agony lasted another two hours. There was a rattle in his throat, a twitching in his wasted body. Then the rattle and the gasping came at longer intervals.
>
> ii. 'It is over!' some one said over him.
>
> iii. He caught those words and repeated them in his soul.
>
> iv. 'Death is over,' he said to himself. 'It's no more.' He drew in a breath, stopped midway in the breath, stretched and died. (pp. 69, 70)

Someone is eager to announce the end. Ivan takes the words into his soul. There they are transformed: the 'It' that has pursued him is light. Ivan's question, "What is the right thing?" has been a steadfast search through his relationships for what is life. Through the questioning, he has let go of the things that have kept him away from home. "Death is over." Vanya has come home. Death is over. Vanya has come home.

Letting Go of the Things

Caius to Ivan

Kiseveter's syllogism is true (correct) and the closure effected by its logical structure is an achievement that Ivan prizes in his profession. But the generalization, "All men are mortal," does not respond to the question of justice, Why ought "all men" die? Also, there is no life in the abstraction, "Caius is a man"; there is no memory of a man. Ivan is a man with memories. Why ought Ivan die?

Moments to Memories

We distill moments into memories. "What is past has been saved and rescued by us into the past," writes Frankl.[8] These memories bear no claim to fame or glory; these memories witness to an 'ordinary' life touched with mystery and beauty, as momentary as the perfect snowflake melting on my jacket.

In the moment of death, memories die. Though the aging grandfather tells his grandaughter his memories, he knows she is too young to remember since yesterday is already a sleep away. And so, the treasures found in life are hid in death. But they are not lost. The child remembers her grandfather by her love, the heart of her memories of her moments with him. And she remembers that he told her his memories.

Invalid to In-valid

The invalid must be strong to keep from becoming in-valid, (L. *in*, 'not': *validus*, 'strong').[9] "It is necessary to maintain an attitude of everyday banality," Aries writes. "On this condition, the sick man may be able to maintain his morale. He needs all his strength to do this."[10] Though Ivan sees his personal and professional life by a different light (the light of death), he continues to speak as if he possesses command of his legal and household matters. Self-sufficiency is the boundary beyond which he would not let colleagues or family pass. "He does not give way, he guards his secret suffering."[11] Nevertheless, he is possessed by the hour of his suffering: he is at stake in the hour. Ivan's hour of suffering is also "the hour of the world," writes Buber.[12] How could one alone bear the hour of the world in the hour of personal tragedy?

Ivan is alienated from the hour of the world because he is alienated even from his own family. "He saw that no one felt for him because no one even wished to grasp his position."[13] Yet his illness makes him dependent on them for their care. But how to care for a self-sufficient man? He is "simply ill," they tell him, "need only keep quiet...follow the doctor's orders...." He hears the self-sufficiency he has bounded his life by parrotting him in the voices and manner of his family. In the hour of his need, the family members 'make' him an invalid while invalidating his experience of suffering and dying.

Dis-ease to Disease

"For Ivan Ilyitch, his illness is suddenly a case that has a separate existence and must have a name. What name? It is up to the doctor to say it, and then he will know whether or not it is serious," Aries writes.[14] Ivan knows his illness as suffering (dis-ease); the doctor knows Ivan's illness as organic malfunction (disease).[15] The doctor has a name for the malfunction. There is no name for the suffering. So the name of the disease puts the dis-ease in perspective. Is Ivan seriously ill? Will he get better? Or is he terminally ill? These are the "real question[s] of life and death"[16]—the questions of dis-ease which the diagnosis of disease should answer.

Pain to Despair

Ivan experiences pain as an absence of all that made him satisfied in life in a way which puts him in question. The presence of pain is cruelty, punishment, senselessness. His response to pain—despair, is a recognition that he is not the center of existence, that the center to which he had drawn all things is empty. Ivan despairs of God, because he despairs of himself. Marcel writes, "Despair asserts that God has withdrawn himself from me, asserts a reality I do not possess:"[17] there is nothing apart from God. Yet Ivan finds nothing good in himself or in the world he has fashioned. Deceit is at the very heart of it. How could God dwell there?

Help to Hope

The needy master

The hour flows through Ivan in the way he lives the hour.[18] Gentle and honest is the hour of his greatest suffering when his servant, Gerasim, is near. With Gerasim, he does not mask his need because Gerasim is one who recognizes him in his need. Levinas writes, "To recognize the Other is to recognize a hunger. To recognize the Other is to give. But it is to give to the master, to the lord, to him who approaches as "You" in the dimension of height."[19] For Gerasim, the hour of the world, Ivan's hour of suffering, and his own hour with Ivan are one. "We shall all of us die so why should I grudge a little trouble?"[20]

Hope is a promise of help

The "need for some hope illustrates that life hangs on fragile threads of promise from one person to another."[21] Though Ivan's doctor does not name the disease (that remains a silent battle inside Ivan), there is a "thread of promise" in the doctor's "serious, but not . . . hopeless face," and in his word, a "chance" of recovery.[22] The minister, however, gives Ivan the "hope of life"[23] in the Sacrament—the assurance that God dwells with him through the atoning death of Christ, the assurance that life is worth living. Anchored in this hope, the doctor's "chance" becomes Ivan's plan for surgery and after, a commitment to live through pain.

Judgment to Mercy

Ivan had judged his wife and family according to his judgment of himself. Set free from self-condemnation to die in peace, he longs to free them from his condemnation. However, even as he entrusts his death to God, he entrusts their life together to Him, for he could not say the word, forgive. "He tried to say 'forgive,' but said 'forego.' "[24] The tears and grief of his wife and son 'speak' their forgiveness and love at parting. Would they ponder his last word to them? Would they forgo the things of life to find the meaning of life? Would they treasure each other?

All Moments to the Last Moment

And calmest thoughts come round us—as, of leaves
Budding,—fruit ripening in stillness,—autumn suns

Smiling at eve upon the quiet sheaves,—
Sweet Sappho's cheek,—a sleeping infant's breath,—
The gradual sand that through an hour-glass runs,—
A woodland rivulet,—a Poet's death.

—John Keats[25]

The meaning of the last moment, the moment of forgiveness, does not suffer change even though time passes. Suffering is not strong enough to take away joy and peace. Suffering which questioned Ivan's joy and peace in the beginning, has become the place and time of his joy and peace. For if Ivan could not find joy and peace in suffering, where could he find It?

CHAPTER 8

PAULINE ERICKSON: ONE WITH THE OTHER

He doeth much that loveth much.

—Thomas à Kempis

On "Pauline's Diary": The Patient Speaks

In 1971 when she was twenty-one, Pauline Erickson was diagnosed as having pulmonary hypertension, a disease that slowly destroys arteries in the lungs causing heart failure. It wasn't until ten years later that the disease became the central fact of her life as she began to require oxygen supply most of the time. She died while waiting for a heart-lung transplant. Pauline recorded her experience of illness in a diary which was published in part by her husband, Rev. Brian Erickson.[1] Pauline's diary attests to the meaning of suffering and hope, the meaning of one with the other.

Self-pity

How is self-pity honorable?

> December 2, 1980. I always had felt self-pity was a despicable feeling—but no more. True, to be healthy we cannot linger with that feeling. But every one of us has in our lifetime come face-to-face with self-pity. For some it is extremely transient. For others it overstays its welcome. But for some self-pity is an honorable step toward becoming a total person. (p. 12)

111

No longer healthy, we pity ourselves. Yet self-pity is not despicable, at least for a time, because self-pity is a way of seeking what is lost. We are lost. When we are well, we are embodied in our plans for our future: we make plans as if tomorrow belonged to us, and we, to tomorrow. So our future is as familiar to us as our past and present. When disease strikes, however, we no longer belong in this structure of achievements and expectations. We no longer belong in this world. The body structures our world, lending the room and the bed its sickness; we dwell in a sickroom, a sickbed. But in a sense we no longer belong to our body. We are emptied of all that is familiar. We are a victim of disease. This thought strikes panic in us for the language remembers what we had forgotten: a victim (L. *victima*) was a 'beast of sacrifice'[2] in Roman times. We are bewildered. We had been at ease in the body of our daily life, heeding the calling of clocks and appetite and busy-ness. Nothing calls us anymore; neither the past nor the future, nor clocks or appetite or busy-ness. Dis-ease banishes ease. Self-pity fills the vacuum. Self-pity is the fullness of our sorrow when we are emptied of routine.

Pain

Where is God in the experience of pain? How do we prevent the comfort of God's presence? How do we work through grief?

> December 2, 1980. I want to say, God, where are you? But I know you're here with me and that you care. But I hurt. I need you and you're here—but I still hurt. Shouldn't your presence comfort me more than it does? What am I lacking? Perhaps I have to fully work through my grief before the comfort. (p. 12)

The mystery of pain dwells in the roots of our nature, in the history of our bones. If pain were a problem, complete before us, we could attack the problem and solve it. But we try to evade pain. Lindell, a Lutheran missionary, writes that pain cannot be evaded by "perfume, roses, soft music, as when the undertaker gave me a handful of rose petals to scatter upon the top of a casket at the grave in place of dirt, as I came to pronounce the fateful words of God: 'You are dust and to dust you shall return.' "[3] Yet the cry of pain, "I hurt," inclines us towards the face of God. Never did God seem nearer, or further away. "In Him, we live and move and have our being."[4] The breath of life that is in us is His breath. Our hurt is His hurt. So we look to the omnipotence of God. This is the nearness, and the distance, of God. And we look to the image of His Son dying on a cross. This is the nearness, and the distance, of God. To look to God is to focus our wanderings into the pathway of a journey. The pathway reorients us to our past, our present, our future. We no longer pity ourselves: we grieve. The Latin word for grieve, *grávure*, means to "charge with a load, burden, weigh down."[5] Not only do we look back and mourn the loss of the unity of will and action, the oneness of spirit and body. We take up the burden of journeying while being bound in pain. Our conflict becomes our comfort: pain cannot destroy us. The mystery of pain beckons us to search for abundant life.

Blessings

We are blessed in the measure we are willing to receive blessing.

> January 1981. Dear God, thank you for giving me the tools to see my life beyond my illness, in spite of my illness, and the ability to love life even though I am unhealthy and may die in the not-too-distant future. Granted, I still get jealous of healthy, productive people—but not despairingly so, for there are things in my life I feel very blessed to have. (p. 12)

Illness is not everything. The pain of illness reminds us of our dying body. But this pain also reminds us of our blessings, the good things in life that we often take for granted. We see the dew on the roses on a sunlit morning. We hear the laughter of children at play. A smile delights us. A sunbeam intrigues us. These "small things"[6] nourish our being, giving us food for thought during the long hours of our illness. We usually measure life by physical activity and productivity: working, shopping, exercising, eating, playing, studying. So we feel jealous of all exuberantly healthy people we meet. But we slowly learn that our attitude transforms small joys—including the busy joys of those around us—into lasting treasures. We are blessed.

Changing

i.   *The daily life of illness is a struggle towards unachievable expectations.*
ii. *The daily life of illness is an acceptance of the gift of the day.*

> i. March 9, 1982. I look around at this world and feel sad—sad because I'm not "intensely aware" of my life and the beauty of it; of its miraculous nature. I've read that when one faces death, one becomes radiantly alive. Something is wrong here. With all the things going on in this world, all the things needing to be done, all the people suffering, I "should" be focusing on something besides TV.
>
> ii. I do want to leave something to the world, but I have so little energy. And most of the energy I have to spare is directed to Brian. I love him; I'm going to miss him; I want to be with him every waking moment until I die. Yes, I can hear the birds chirping and smell the flowers. It's wonderful to be alive. (p. 13)

Searching for abundant life, we expect change in ourselves. We are saddened by the reality of our daily existence. Disease seemed to strike us down in a moment: illness lasts a long time; long enough to live with it, long enough to die. Each day of living is a day of dying. And every way of living is a way of dying. "Pain and death," Lindell writes, "are something we do."[7] How we 'do' pain and death—our daily life—becomes our work for those we love. Even so, times are. We remember the illness at times; we are discouraged and im-patient. And we forget the illness at times; we live through it. Through it all, we are changing: we are the world in pain. All that suffers is ours, not only as a way of having, but as a way of being—a way of doing. Pain is our valley and hope is our mountain, and silence surrounds all and fills all. And we respond to the song of the birds with wonder-ful attention. Each of our days is an invitation to live as though it were our dying day.

Giving

To live is to give. What can we give that means something?

> March 13, 1982. Dear God, please help me to live long enough so I can help and touch more people's lives. I am your servant. Please help me to truly relinquish all foolish claims to be in control of my life! I want my life to mean something, and it only can when I is i, and i let you be rightfully in charge.(p. 13)

To be the world in pain is to quell I, to be i: one of one and one and one. As one, even one, the experience of illness is transformed from 'Why must I suffer and die?' to 'Now is my turn to suffer and die.' We resist the I that wells up in resentment to the illness, and therefore, to the kindness that is community. We cannot understand how pain serves to accomplish God's purpose of the good. But each of us remembers how the life of one in pain gave us courage to continue our journey. We help each other. Each life is a gift of life to Life.

Transcending Captivity

Escapism leads to depression. Thankfulness for faith, love, enables acceptance.

> April 2, 1982. When I become "seriously" ill, will I continually be depressed because my little mental game can no longer bolster me? After a bit of trepidation, I can answer a hopeful no. . .I have my belief and faith in God, who gives me courage and, more importantly, love. I love Brian. Our love is everlasting. I have the love of my family, the love of my friends. I am truly blessed. I have been to the mountaintop. Life is beautiful: it hurts but I can leave it. (p. 14)

"Experience is not so much an absorbing into oneself of something as a straining oneself towards something."[8] Experience is an openness to more experience, even when the typical experience of physical movement is so difficult that our own body becomes an object for us. We will that the body move, but the body resists our intention. When we try to draw the hand towards the face to wash or feed ourself, we experience the weakness of damaged muscles. The hand never reaches the face. It is incapable of doing what we ask. We bolster our hope for physical recovery by testing our endurance each day: we sit up for an hour; we walk a few steps. Though we persist, our body remains an obstacle in the gestalt of daily life. Our will must be actualized through something other than physical movement. Experiencing the body as a captivity, we look to "the shining of that veiled mysterious light."[9] Always, at the end, there is no end. The body, after all, is not the source or limit of our being.

Hope

i.   *The meaning of hope is bound up with the events of Easter.*
ii.   *Illness is a time to prepare for Easter in our own lives.*

> i. April 1982. Happy Easter! This Sunday is such a day of jubilation—Christ lives! In the mode of the sermon I heard today, this weekend is a microcosm of life. Friday—despair, desolation, heartbreak, hell, and death; Saturday— loneliness, grief; Sunday—joy, happiness, life anew!
>
> ii. Brian, if you must face my death, remember Friday. It will be hell. But Saturday you will be able to live through— because of God's love you can do it. (We have something so special—I hope it lasts much longer. But if not, we have had 10 beautiful years.) Sunday, Brian, you will be happy. You will always miss me, but that does not mean missing out on life. (p. 14)

"Remember Friday. It will be hell." All through life there is the pain caused by the thought of death because we yearn to live on. Buytendijk writes that an heroic attitude to death bypasses the nature of pain and death. Heroism denies our personal existence: we, too, must die. Weeping bears witness to our personal existence. When we weep, we stand outside what is happening to us. But we cannot always weep. So we surrender to pain as a condition of life. We experience the "whole extent" of its destruction.[10] We experience our mortality. Thousands of years ago, the psalmist wrote,

> The days of our years are threescore and ten;
> and if by reason of strength they be fourscore years,
> Yet is their strength labour and sorrow;
> for it is soon cut off, and we fly away.[11]

We know life one day at a time. Would we know the grief and loneliness of Saturday if our heart did not break on Friday? Would we know the joy of Sunday if we did not journey through Friday and Saturday? We know that a seed lives again as a seedling. Is our destiny less than that of a seed? In humility, we hope for the joy of Sunday. There can be no humility—no hope—except through the temptation to despair: the humility of hope is "a response to the infinite Being to whom it is conscious of owing everything that it has and upon whom it cannot impose any condition whatsoever without scandal."[12] Friday. . . Saturday. . . Sunday. . ."You will miss me but that does not mean missing out on life." Hope is stronger than death.

Hope for Tomorrow

What are we asking when we ask God to heal us?

> April 1982. Dear God, I do not want to die. Please help me to hang in there until (and after!) the surgery. I adamantly believe in your power to heal people. If it's your will, please heal me. God, don't take me from Brian, not yet. (p. 14)

A funeral cortege slowly drove toward the cemetery. Impatient motorists sped past the procession. A few motorists drove slowly behind and so became a part of the procession. At the cemetery gate, they continued on their way. We do not want to die. We who race against death do not want to die.

We who acknowledge death do not want to die. We who are ill do not want to die. We who are healed do not want to die. We do not want to die yet.

Peace

i.   *Need to be alone means to be with a loved one, with a book, with God.*
ii. *Need to seek peace takes precedence over other needs.*

> i. April 29,1982. Am I dying? Yes, I feel it. Also the aloneness (of my own doing), except for Brian. I want to be by myself and meditate. Brian gave me an excellent book by Meister Eckhart, a 13th-century Christian mystic. It has made me feel so inadequate, but I feel I am getting deeper in my soul and becoming more in tune with God.
>
> ii. I hope I will thank, either verbally, or by letter, the wonderfully caring, supportive, and love-filled friends I have here. But right now I have to focus more on my inner life and peace.(p. 14)

Whenever we try to understand ourself, "the whole perceptible world comes too, and with it comes the others who are caught in it."[13] Even when we are deeply alone, companions come along—other travelers, present and past, whose words speak to us. Thus, the fabric of our human experience draws us deeper into ourself. Gustave Thibon writes, "If you fly away from yourself, your prison will run with you and will close in because of the wind of your flight; if you go deep down into yourself, it will disappear in paradise."[14] Our paradise is peace in the midst of pain and death. The Latin word for peace, *pacem*, means to make a treaty. Life costs us pain and death. Life gives us peace.

Hope for Today

i.   *Concern centers on others.*
ii. *Reflection leads to deeper understanding.*
iii. *God suffers.*
iv. *Life and death intertwine.*
v.   *Life is an individual journey.*

i. May 22, 1982. I'm alive now. Please help me make the most of it, Lord. I do not want to spend what might be my last days bitter, depressed, or sullen. I want to leave Brian with good remembrances of me.

ii. I do not seem to laugh anymore. Is it because I get out of wind, or is the great expert on death and dying having trouble coping? Whatever the reason, I want to leave with a smile on my face.

iii. My theology, please don't desert me now. It would be much easier to be a radical right-winger—to say this is all God's will. But I believe that God doesn't cause suffering and that many times God doesn't interfere. Thus, if I am dying, let God's tears be enough. It is enough.

iv. God, please make my heart less heavy. Is the burden death, or is it lethargy from illness?

v. God, I want to be like Eckhart and say, "Your will be done." But I don't want to die. I just want to talk to you about my tears. (p. 15)

We say, "I'm alive now," with feeling, as we struggle to move, to breathe. For life is more than the body yet bound to the body. We do not have the stamina to laugh and to weep—we find almost no avenue for expression through our body. In this moment of tension between life and death, this last moment, we hear no trumpets sounding. Only "I'm alive now," a pronouncement of the existence of one, an exclamation that fades like a sigh. Our life, still recognizable to others as this dying body, is known to God as this "dying heart."[15] This dying heart, so heavy within us. And pain in this heart, which made the breach between will and action, begins to make one again. "For where was my heart to flee for refuge from my heart?" asks Augustine.[16] We do not want a sullen heart, or bitter, or depressed. We want a heart like the heart of God, a heart that is willing to die. Yet we struggle to be born into a life of illness, to be born to die. For still the day calls us, calls us to join in the celebration of life. And still, the celebration re-calls us, re-calls us to the remembrance of our death. And still, so still, the day of our remembrance. Death is silent still.

The Struggle to be Born into a Life of Illness

Self-pity is Honorable as a Step Away from Self-pity

Self-pity is capitulation to illness. In fighting against capitulation, we learn what we are fighting for. David Cornelius describes his fight against capitulation when he experienced bone cancer at age eight.[17] His description, written in high school, highlights three moments in the experience of self-pity as an honorable step away from self-pity:

i.   *the medical diagnosis and response to the diagnosis;*
ii.   *help to live through the diagnosis and response to the help;*
iii. *out of (ii) a third moment emerges, acceptance of illness as life for 'me.'*

> i. The staff at Egleston found the cancer and although they said I was lucky to have it diagnosed so quickly, I didn't feel lucky. There was a possibility, they said, that my left arm would have to go. Why me? What had I done to deserve this?
>
> ii. At Egleston, a nurse came and helped me to write a list of all the good things should worse come to worst in the pending operation. Before I realized what was happening, I was feeling both happy and relieved.
>
> iii. She helped me to discover how fortunate I was that my writing hand wouldn't be affected and that at my young age adjustments would be much easier. Then the cards started coming. Although I found solace in each of hundreds that I received, one in particular filled me with wonder. It told me to read Psalm 6. I read the whole passage but it was verse two that gave me comfort:
>
> Have mercy upon me, O Lord; for I am weak: O Lord, heal me; for my bones are vexed.
>
> I had the odd sensation that the David of long ago had written this verse just for me, a small child with bone cancer who wanted to be healed and needed God's mercy. (p. 8)

The medical diagnosis brought a response of self-pity, "I didn't feel lucky... Why me? What had I done to deserve this?" The experience of self-pity became a concerted fight against self-pity through the help of a nurse. David responded by "feeling both happy and relieved." This response was an acknowledgement that "she helped me to discover how fortunate I was." Within his being was the possibility of living with illness. He was also supported by his friends who assured him of comfort, love and faith. Within his community was the possibility of living with illness.

The Pain of Illness

The pain of illness is loss.

The possibility of amputation held out a slim possiblity of not-amputation. David clung to this possibility.

> After a chaotic week of testing, a surgeon informed me that a crucial biopsy would be done the next day during which the decision would be made as to whether or not they would immediately amputate my arm. The next morning, nervous and in a fog of sedation, I saw the operating light, its cold steel gleaming down on me before I went under.
> When I came to, my heart leapt! I could feel my arm! It was still there.

During the surgery, there was one who was praying, keeping vigil at the bedside, the first one to see the truth, the one to bear away the possibility.

> Then I looked over at my mother. The expression on her face told me the hard truth. Suddenly I knew I had been wrong. My mind had tricked me with 'phantom pain.' My arm was gone. That quote from Psalms flashed through my mind:
> "Have mercy upon me, O Lord," and I wondered why such a merciful God would let this happen.
> I was lost, afraid and struggling for something to help me cope. Mom was there. At that dark time she was the only constant in my life.

At that "dark time", in the depths of the experience of the loss of a part of himself, David relied on his mother to be the "constant" in his life. She was there with him. It was all she could do. It was enough. As her gesture of grief bears away the possibility, her gesture of love sustains the days of loss.

The pain of illness is bearing the grief as hope.

When David describes his mother's gesture of hope that opens up new possibilities for living, he speaks first of "we," then of "Mother" or "I." This was the time of a mutual venture.

> One day we walked through the hospital garden. It was spring and all the dogwoods stood against the fence in full bloom; squirrels were running around and birds were calling from the trees. Although, I admit, the garden was small and simple, my mother's words of praise brought out its beauty. She would point out something and proclaim what a wonder it was. Through her joyous eyes, I could see all of the wonders with which God had filled the garden.
>
> That day, we made a pact to see the garden every time we visited the hospital later on for my treatments, so that I would have happy memories to combat the sad ones.

The quiet acceptance of the inevitability of return for chemotherapy treatments meshes with quiet gratitude for the inevitability of the return of the seasons. Winter, too, is a season of hope.

We Find Refuge in Blessings

> I thank God Mom was there. On all our visits to the hospital, she never gave up. It must have been hard on her but again she helped me turn to the garden as a refuge. We stopped entering through the cold front doors of the hospital and started slipping past the small gate into the garden and through the back doors.

The place of refuge was a secret happiness that David would not have known had it not been so very near the place of suffering; a happiness he might have missed had his mother not shared her sight.

Each of Our Days is an Invitation to Live as though it were Our Dying Day

David had fought against capitulation to illness. He had fought for life.

> Then, slowly, a strange desire welled up in me. When I reflected on my life previous to the operation, all I could find was an ordinary boy living an ordinary life—no great accomplishments and no great downfalls. I saw my life now as better, and I decided against staying just level. My grades got better. I joined the band and discovered writing. I found that after going through the operation and chemotherapy, and dealing with my hair loss, I had gained a new self. I started actively living my life—trying to make the best of each and every day. (p. 9) .

Self-pity is a memory, a shed image. Each new day is a possibility. David shows us that something must die to nourish the growth of something else. His story ends with his new beginning.[18]

However, Pauline's illness was one of continual deterioration. Her times of reflection were not about pain or illness but in pain, in illness towards death. Pauline struggled to live fully though she could scarcely breathe. What was her new beginning? She knew life by her love.

To Live is to Give

The presence of one who is loved is the most precious gift of all. For example, Joni Eareckson Tada, who is quadrapelegic, tells how her husband becomes her hands for two hours each week as he tends the garden following her instructions.[19] Could she give as much? To live is already to give. Just listening to her makes one happy. Only Joni could give her thankfulness, her love for Jesus, her humor, her art;

just as only Pauline could give her struggle, her strength, her faith, her hope.

The Body, After All, is not the Source or the Limit of Our Being

God doth not need
Either man's work or his own gifts; who best
Bear his mild yoke, they serve Him best. His state
Is kingly. Thousands at his bidding speed
And post o'er land and ocean without rest.
They also serve who only stand and wait.

—John Milton[20]

Frankl wrote that man's last freedom is to choose his attitude, to choose his own way.[21] For Milton, his own way was God's way for him. He served God by bearing his blindness, by taking for his "ownmost being-in-the-world"[22] an alien place, a place of certain struggle, certain hardship, certain limitation. The pain of blindness "[did] not incapacitate his life as a person."[23] In his blindness, he gave the world "When I Consider How My Light is Spent."

Hope is Stronger than Death

Hope is the acceptance of blessings not yet received.

My sister, Joy, suffered from a debilitating bone disease because of kidney failure and dialysis. Though she could barely walk, she was a full-time student in Education. The time came for her to be a student-teacher. How could she teach children when she could barely walk, when every movement hurt? She prayed for healing. One day, this prayer would be answered and she would know again freedom of movement. But this day, the first day of life in her chosen profession, she awoke with the familiar pain. She wept. Dad comforted her with the promises of God. "God has something good for you there," he said, "but you can't know unless you go." They prayed together. Joy chose to go. The first provision was evident from the car—no stairway into the school. Dad walked with her to the door and opened it for her. Thus far he could go with her and no farther. He stood in the entry and watched her walk away. But God was with her all the way. In the Principal's Office, she met Sister Dorothy, who was also the only teacher as the school would close a year hence when the current grade 4/5 students would graduate to another school.

Sister Dorothy's sister was suffering from bone cancer. How deeply she understood Joy's pain! She helped Joy plan lessons that made the most of teaching possibilities within a limited range of teacher movements. Most of all, she taught Joy what it means to live a life of care with children for whom one is responsible as teacher. The children shared in responsible care. When a classmate was ill, they prayed for his recovery. And they were determined to make Joy a teacher. When the faculty consultant left after observing a lesson, they asked, "Are you a teacher yet?" Joy received her accreditation for teaching.

Joy lived through the pain of that experience in the promise, "Lo, I am with you always, even to the close of the age."[24] What she gave to Sister Dorothy and the children cannot be measured. What Sister Dorothy and the children gave to her cannot be measured. Joy and Sister Dorothy became friends for life.

Hope is the longing for healing.

What are we asking when we ask God to heal us? Health for Pauline was freedom to breathe with ease. No longer was the sky the limit. The limit was so close to her being, so near to her heart. Yet her diary discloses that the healing she received, though not physical, was real.

In Shelley's poem, "To a Skylark," dwells a deep sense of this meaning of healing.

> We look before and after,
> And pine for what is not;
> Our sincerest laughter

With some pain is fraught;
Our sweetest songs are those
that tell of saddest thought.

Yet if we could scorn
Hate, and pride, and fear;
If we were things born
Not to shed a tear,
I know not how thy joy ever
should come near.[25]

Pauline could hear life's poem in the birdsong because her life was the refrain. She accepted each day as life for her, she loved life unconditionally. This acceptance was a question as these lines from Shelley's poem are a question. Through sorrow, could we learn what is joy? Through illness, what is health? Through death, what is life?

Hope is the acceptance of what we cannot understand.

"I want to leave with a smile on my face."[25] Pauline gave God her tears. God gave her a smile. How could there be a smile on her face if there were no smile in her heart? And how could there be a smile in her heart if her heart were not reconciled to smile? Reconciled to God, the Giver of life, and the Giver of life in death.

We bear the grief of death as hope.

This way that Pauline walked, was the way of one. Yet, through her individual journey, she was bound more closely to her community, those who were willing to suffer and rejoice with her on their individual journeys. Pauline did not want the meaning of her life to be the pain her death caused her family and friends. She left those she loved with a grief that could be borne as hope because of her hope, "Sunday. . .you will be happy."

Life Gives Us Peace

If I could paint a poem of peace, I would paint a summer evening at sunset, the air still warm, and sweet with the smell of clover. And there, at the edge of the farmer's field, *Scandia*, the church my grandfather helped to build. There I am, too, with my family, watching through the windows as the sun glows the grain and the graves into gold. There in the sanctuary, labour and sorrow are beautified as worship and praise before the altar of God. There in the midst, a place set apart, a poem of peace.

CHAPTER 9

DOCTOR RIEUX: ONE FOR THE OTHER

Nothing in life is to feared,
It is only to be understood.

—Marie Curie

On *The Plague*: The Doctor Speaks

Albert Camus received the Nobel Prize for Literature in 1957 for *The Plague*.[1] In his acceptance speech, he said,

> For more than twenty years of an insane history, hopelessly lost like all the men of my generation in the convulsions of time, I have been supported by one thing: by the hidden feeling that to write today was an honor because this activity was a commitment—and a commitment not only to write. Specifically, in view of my powers and my state of being, it was a commitment to bear, together with all those who were living through the same history, the misery and hope we shared.[2]

Plague is a life of misery, and hope. The novel, *The Plague*, describes a profound test of human being, a situation that relentlessly requires, in Levinas' words, the "chosen one" to be "for the other."[3] The novel is set in Oran, which Camus describes as a large French port on the Algerian coast, where he lived for a year and experienced plague. Doctor Rieux, the narrator in the novel, is a citizen of Oran. Tarrou, his friend, is a visitor to Oran who is compelled to stay in the city when the gates are closed because of plague. Doctor Castel researches for an anti-plague serum. Paneloux is the priest.

129

The Fact of the Doctor's Diagnosis

i.   *Pity satisfies when it is tied to useful action.*
ii. *Hope resides in the person of the doctor.*
iii. *The doctor's evidence dispels hope.*
iv. *Grief takes the place of hope.*

> i. "Have some pity, doctor!" It was Mme Loret, mother of the chambermaid at Tarrou's hotel, who made the appeal. An unnecessary appeal; of course he had pity. But what purpose could it serve? He had to telephone, and soon the ambulance could be heard clanging down the street. (At first the neighbors used to open windows and watch. Later they promptly shut them.) Then came a second phase of conflict, tears and pleadings—abstraction, in a word. In those fever-hot, nerve-ridden sickrooms crazy scenes took place. But the issue was always the same. The patient was removed. Then Rieux, too, could leave.
>
> ii. ...every evening was like that evening when he was called in for Mme Loret's daughter. He was shown into a small apartment decorated with fans and artificial flowers. The mother greeted him with a faltering smile. "Oh, I do hope it's not the fever everyone's talking about."
>
> iii. Lifting the coverlet and chemise, he gazed in silence at the red blotches on the girl's thighs and stomach, the swollen ganglia. After one glance the mother broke into shrill, uncontrollable cries of grief.
>
> iv. And every evening mothers wailed thus, with a distraught abstraction, as their eyes fell on those fatal stigmata on limbs and bellies; every evening hands gripped Rieux's arms, there was a rush of useless words, promises, and tears; every evening the nearing tocsin of the ambulance provoked scenes as vain as every form of grief. (p. 54)

Pity is useless. Grief is useless. Neither pity nor grief changes the situation. Yet we pity. We grieve. Pity and grief change us, and we see the situation differently. "Everybody knows that pestilences have a way of recurring in the world; yet somehow we find it hard to believe in ones that crash down on our heads from a blue sky."[4] We know that pestilences scourge faceless masses. But these faces are familiar, these lives are precious; the chambermaid at Tarrou's hotel is Mme Loret's daughter.

The fear of plague turns us cold, colors us grey. So we shut our windows against it. Yet, the cold greyness of the fear of plague calls us to suffer pity, to suffer grief; to suffer our human being. The cold greyness of the fear of plague brings us to live what we cannot reason out. Therefore, we pity Mme Loret for her daughter's sake. And we grieve for Mme Loret's daughter for her mother's sake. Through their suffering, we remember that there are no faceless masses, only families and separated families who suffer and rejoice as we do. This, too, is life. And life is dear to us.

The Doctor Finds Solace

How does the doctor experience pity when it is not tied to useful action?

> One grows out of pity when it's useless. And in this feeling that his heart had slowly closed in on itself, the doctor found a solace, his only solace, for the almost unendurable burden of his days. This, he knew, would make his task easier, and therefore he was glad of it. When he came home at two in the morning and his mother was shocked at the blank look he gave her, she was deploring precisely the sole alleviation Rieux could then experience. (p. 54)

How long can we pity? How long can we grieve? How long before our tears break one last time?

> All streams run to the sea,
> but the sea is not full;
> to the place where the streams flow,
> there they flow again.
> All things are full of weariness
> a man cannot utter it.[5]

With a "blank look," a weary doctor asks, "Why?" Camus writes, "everything begins in that weariness tinged with amazement." The weariness comes "at the end of the acts of a mechanical life, but at the same time it inaugurates the impulse of consciousness."[6] Weariness inaugurates the impulse of consciousness of community. We all alike must suffer. We all alike must die. We all alike must ask, "Why?" The weariness, like amazement, is pervasive. "All streams run to the sea but the sea is not full."

The Meanings of Being a Doctor

i. *Achievement is one of the meanings of being a doctor.*
ii. *Death is one of the meanings of being a doctor.*
iii. *The doctor feels personally responsible for death.*
iv. *Suffering defeats the doctor.*

> i. "When I entered this profession, I did it 'abstractly,' so to speak; because it meant a career like another, one that young men often aspire to. Perhaps, too, because it was particularly difficult for a workman's son, like myself.
>
> ii. And then I had to see people die. Do you know that there are some who *refuse* to die? Have you ever heard a woman scream 'Never!' with her last gasp? Well, I have. And then I saw that I could never get hardened to it. I was young then, and I was outraged by the whole scheme of things, or so I thought. Subsequently I grew more modest. Only, I've never managed to get used to seeing people die. That's all I know."
>
> iii. [Tarrou is speaking]. . . "I now can picture what this plague must mean for you."
> "Yes. A never ending defeat."
>
> iv. Tarrou stared at the doctor for a moment, then turned and tramped heavily toward the door. Rieux followed him and was almost at his side when Tarrou, who was staring at the floor, suddenly said; "Who taught you all this, doctor?"
> The reply came promptly: "Suffering." (p. 73)

The doctor[7] says that the high profile, respectable status of the medical profession calls young people to its practice.

The medical profession is a challenge. However, the challenge of the medical profession is only partially fulfilled through the challenge of academic competition or the challenge of brilliant diagnosis. The fundamental challenge of the medical profession is the ill and dying patients for whom the doctor cares. The doctor cannot be trained to make an adequate response to this challenge: the doctor learns to respond to this challenge by living through many difficult experiences. Reflecting on these experiences, the doctor tries to overcome what he perceives to be personal or professional deficiencies.

Yet we must not separate the personal and professional aspects of the practise of medicine as if the doctor could be 'entirely professional' or 'too personal.' The profession of medicine involves the person, the person is mediated through the profession. So death is not a "never ending defeat"; the doctor, too, must die. The doctor says that he experiences life's events with the patient, including death. The doctor can help the ill and dying to the limit of his or her professional care. Suffering is the meeting-place, the place where doctor and patient share the ache of all human existence. Suffering is the meeting-place, the place where doctor and patient share the hope of all human existence. The doctor says, "There is no cure now but there will be someday."

To Have a Heart for Healing and No Cure

i.   *The doctor diagnoses disease in order to cure. What is it like for the doctor when there is no cure?*

ii. *To have a heart means to endure, to start each day anew.*

> i. He knew that, over a period whose end he could not glimpse, his task was no longer to cure but to diagnose, detect, to see, to describe, to register, and then condemn— that was his present function. Sometimes a woman would clutch his sleeve, crying shrilly: "Doctor, you'll save him, won't you?" But he wasn't there for saving life; he was there to order a sick man's evacuation. How futile was the hatred he saw on faces then! "You haven't a heart!" a woman told him on one occasion. She was wrong; he had one.

ii. It saw him through his twenty-hour day, when he hourly watched men dying who were meant to live. It enabled him to start anew each morning. He had just enough heart for that, as things were now. How could that heart have sufficed for saving life? (p. 101)

Neither the populace nor the medical community understood plague. People died within a few days with the plague because early indicators were not recognized, and Doctor Castel was attempting to develop an anti-plague serum as the plague raged on. Therefore, the experience of plague in the novel is analogous to the diagnosis and treatment of some types of cancer today.

The doctor speaks the word: "Cancer." How much heart does a doctor need to pronounce the word, to live that eternal moment with the patient? That moment that robs the future of its promise, the past of its fulfillment, the present of its living action. All is reflection now. But there is not time for reflection. All is regret now. But there is not time for regret. We must get to the business of dying. Through the thick fog of all the possibilities and the never-to-be-achieved, the patient acknowledges the verdict. Does the doctor share the numbness? Does the doctor have a heart? "Yes," says the doctor, but is there enough heart to cope with anything beyond that word that ends the day? Is there enough heart to return to hospital rounds and office appointments and the appointment to choose wallpaper for the living room at home? Is there enough heart to continue to live as if the day had not died the moment—the eternal moment—the word was spoken? How can there be enough heart? And yet, the doctor and the patient do continue as if that eternal moment did not hold sway.

Life and the Doctor of Death

i. *The doctor who brings grief is the doctor of death.*
ii. *The doctor is also made of dust.*
iii. *The doctor restrains his pity when he is with the patient.*

i. Before the plague he was welcomed as a savior. He was going to make them right with a couple of pills or an injection, and people took him by the arm on his way to the sickroom. Flattering, but dangerous. Now, on the contrary, he came accompanied by soldiers, and they had to hammer on the door with rifle-butts before the family would open it.

ii. They would have liked to drag him, drag the whole human race, with them to the grave.

iii. Yes, it was quite true that men can't do without their fellow men; that he was as helpless as these unhappy people and he, too, deserved the same faint thrill of pity that he allowed himself once he had left them. (p. 101)

Doctor Rieux continually dealt with the consequence of plague: death. The doctor became the symbol of death to the families who could not escape the presence of plague in their homes: they could not escape the doctor of death. Consequently, the doctor came to represent the patients' disease. In their awesome sorrow, the patients' families forgot the comforting presence of the doctor during other trying days, days when illness meant a sensible prescription: rest in bed, drink plenty of fluids, take one tablet twice daily.

The doctor controls the emotion of pity in order to live the life of pity. But who pities the doctor? The doctor himself needs a physician. "Is there no balm in Gilead? Are there no physicians there?"[8] The doctor shares with the priesthood the profession of giving. But the doctor does not necessarily share the minister's source of strength. The minister offers salvation. The doctor offers "some good life" during a difficult time. "Some good life," says the doctor, means to return to work, for one; to continue education, for an other; to travel, for an other. "Some good life" means that death occurs sooner for these than for the general population. "Some good life" means treating the disease, reducing suffering, or helping the patient cope. "Some good life" means a gift, even if only a respite in the face of death. And, "some good life" is the doctor's reward when death comes. "Some good life" is the physician's healing balm.

The Doctor Fights for Life

i.   *A new day.*
ii. *A time to fight.*
iii. *A time to die.*
iv. *A time to "move back."*

> i. Light was increasing in the ward. The occupants of the other nine beds were tossing about and groaning, but in tones that seemed deliberately subdued. . . Only the child went on fighting with all his little might.
>
> ii. Now and then Rieux took his pulse—less because this served any purpose than as an escape from his utter helplessness—and when he closed his eyes, he seemed to feel its tumult mingling with the fever of his own blood.
>
> iii. And then, at one with the tortured child, he struggled to sustain him with all the remaining strength in his own body.
>
> iv. But, linked for a few moments, the rhythms of their heartbeats soon fell apart, the child escaped him, and again he knew his impotence. Then he released the small, thin wrist and moved back to his place. (p. 112)

Each of us has a place. Regardless of how close the doctor feels to the child, how valiantly he fights against the child's death, the doctor cannot give life. The doctor must keep his place. "Some good life" is given and the doctor and patient make the best of it. "Some good life" is taken. And the doctor is left in his place.

The Doctor Questions All Values

i.   *What do we lose when we die of plague?*
ii. *What do we win when we survive plague?*

> i. Tarrou had died this evening without their friendship's having had time to enter fully into the life of either. Tarrou had "lost the match," as he put it. But what had he, Rieux, won?

ii. No more than the experience of having known plague and remembering it, of having known friendship and remembering it, of knowing affection and being destined one day to remember it. So all a man could win in the conflict between plague and life was knowledge and memories. But Tarrou, perhaps, would have called that winning the match. (p. 148)

"Winning the match" is a fundamental absurdity. All must breathe and hope. In this sense, all must win the match. Had Tarrou "lost the match?" Or is losing the match a fundamental absurdity too? All must suffer and die. In this sense, all must lose the match. Yet death itself "causes us to question all values," the doctor says. What was first in our life? Friendship? Child? Match point? Death reduces the best of life and the worst of life to knowledge and memories—dust and ashes: death buries life. But death also infuses the best of life and the worst of life with hope: death renews life. And each always gives and each always receives, knowledge and memories—and hope. This is the heart of what it means to be a doctor for a patient. This is the heart of pity, (L. *pietas*, 'devotion'),[9] the devotion of care.

The Heart of Pity

Science does not Pity

Eiseley[10] has characterized science as a relentless, searching eye, an eye that sees all and sees nothing. The eye sees all because it is without pity, sees nothing because it is without hope. Eiseley was possessed by the eye. As he walked along the coast of Costabel, the eye saw a starfish dead in the sand. The eye understood that the sea had cast it on the shore and the sand had clogged its pores. The eye saw shell collectors, burdened with sacks. The eye understood that the creatures which did not die in the sand would die in the sacks. And the eye saw the cauldrons of boiling water. The eye understood that the creatures which did not die in the sand or the sacks would die in the water. The eye understood the sea and the death and the greed. For the light in the eye was the observation of survival.

Eiseley walked on. There was one in the distance who gathered starfish and threw them back into the ocean. The eye did not understand the star thrower. And the man possessed by the eye was perplexed.

> Again the eye, the cold world-shrivelling eye, began its inevitable circle in my skull. He is a man, I considered sharply, bringing my thought to rest. The star thrower is a man, and death is running more fleet than he along every seabeach in the world.[11]

Yet the figure of the star thrower at dawn of day evoked memories in the man that the eye did not see, memories of boyhood, disillusion; and the figure of the star thrower evoked speech in the man that the eye could not understand, "I love. . .the things beaten in the strangling surf, the bird, singing, which flies and falls and is not seen again";[12] and the figure of the star thrower evoked action in the man which the eye could not predict, "Silently I sought and picked up a still-living star, spinning it far out into the waves."[13]

Eiseley has described his journey back from observation for its own sake. For him, the eye of (Darwinian) science yielded foregone conclusions: the observation of survival had lost any meaning in the presence of inevitable death.

Science because of Pity

Observation is the keystone of modern medical diagnosis and research. Scientific observation has yielded ways of treating some kinds of cancer, technological advances in dialysis treatment, bone restorative drugs, development in treatment of diabetes, to name a few.[14] These are tremendous advances. Yet illness remains and suffering is increased by some treatments. The patient dies and observation continues. This paradox places us in a question, "Of what rock is the keystone of medical observation quarried?"

The Heart of Pity is "A Sympathy Full of Regret" for "All the Pain."

Doctor Rieux experienced the weariness of pity as the physical and emotional outcome of outrage at the suffering of humanity. His "blank look" was exhausted outrage. Augustine writes, "O foolish man to bear the lot of man so rebelliously."[15] Exhaustion brought the recognition that he could not live in outrage: the "community of suffering"[16] is the "lot of man." Schweitzer writes,

> From this community of suffering I have never tried to withdraw myself. It seemed to me a matter of course that we should all take our share of the burden of pain which lies upon the world."[17]

How does the doctor "take" his or her "share of the burden which lies upon the world" in the context of modern medical science?

The heart of pity is the manner of care.

For Doctor Rieux, the event of diagnostic observation was the official registration of plague in a household enabling the removal of the ill person for the sparing of the family. But the family saw the sparing differently: they would rather care for the one who was ill even if that meant the death of all ("drag the whole human race with them to the grave"). Doctor Rieux was the voice of reason among them. His reason was science; their reason was love. His reason was pity; their reason was despair, and hope.

Doctor Rieux shows how diagnosis can be gentled by the heart of pity even during plague. The old family doctor in *Elsie Venner* by Oliver Wendell Holmes,[18] shows how diagnosis can serve the heart of pity.

> The old doctor was a model for visiting practitioners. He always came into the sickroom with a quiet, cheerful look, as if he had a consciousness he was bringing sure relief with

him. The way a patient snatches his first look at his doctor's face, to see whether he is doomed, whether he is reprieved, whether he is unconditionally pardoned, has really something terrible about it. It is only to be met by an imperturbable mask of serenity, proof against anything and everything in a patient's aspect.[19]

The "sure relief" the old doctor brought was hope. Hope resides in the person of the doctor. The doctor is a "symbol of all that is transferrable from one person to another short of immortality," writes Cousins.[20] In what sense, then, is serenity a mask? Hope is not a resolution of the situation of conflict but a way of living through the conflict. The doctor restrains the expression of pity to perform the action of pity. Schweitzer writes,

> In vain have I tried to train myself to that equanimity which makes it possible for a doctor, in spite of all his sympathy with the sufferings of his patients, to husband, as is desirable, his spiritual and nervous energy.[21]

Schweitzer speaks of the need for disciplined pity, the pity that learns to abide in hope. Hope is the serenity of pity. Truly, serenity is the gift of hope.

The heart of pity is the mortal helping the mortal.

Doctor Rieux was waiting for an anti-plague serum to be developed. The first dose he tried on a child who was dying. The child did not recover. Why did Doctor Rieux give the child the serum? To observe the child's reaction? Because he wanted the child to live? These are the questions of plague, the presence of inevitable death.

> "There wasn't any remission this morning, was there, Rieux?" Rieux shook his head, adding, however, that the child was putting up more resistance than one would have expected. Paneloux, who was slumped against the wall, said in a low voice: "So if he is to die, he will have suffered longer."[22]

Yes, Doctor Rieux wanted the child to live. And yes, he observed the child's reaction. To save the lives of the multitude, he must save this life: the advancement of medicine was the life of the child.

There was no division between the doctor and the observer. The child's death gripped Doctor Rieux and made him 'see'. The child's death was a personal loss to Doctor Rieux, and a personal loss to the multitude. In this sense, death defeats the doctor. He lost the child and the multitude: the need remains. Again, there is one in greatest need.

> "Will you have to start it [anti-plague serum preparation]?" Tarrou asked Castel. The old doctor nodded slowly, with a twisted smile.
> "Perhaps. After all, he put up a surprisingly long resistance."[23]

And the one in greatest need will try the new serum and will suffer—and die, or perhaps, suffer—and live. The multitude waits. Already there is another one in greatest need.

The heart of pity is renewed by death.

Death brings a challenge with defeat, a commitment: this patient must not die in vain. Doctor Scribner, who pioneered the first dialysis unit in North America, writes of the challenge of a patient's death.

> Mr. Saunders had a disease which had totally and irreversibly destroyed his kidneys. They would never function again.
> What to do?. . .We did the only thing we could do. We had an agonizing conversation with Mrs. Saunders and told her to take her husband back home to Spokane where he would die, hopefully without much suffering. . . He died quietly [at home] about two weeks later. . . The emotional impact of this case was enormous on all of us, and I could not stop thinking about it.
> Then one morning about 4:00 A.M. I woke up and groped for a piece of paper and a pencil to jot down the basic idea

of the shunted cannulas which would make it possible for
people like Joe Saunders to dialyze again and again with
the artificial kidney without destroying two blood vessels
each time.[24]

There was no division between the doctor and the
observer. Mr. Saunders' death gripped Doctor Scribner and
made him 'see'. "Pain," writes Levinas, "refers to the joy of
living. Already and henceforth life is loved."[25] "People like
Joe" live. I am like Joe, I needed Scribner's shunt to live. But
the doctor is also like Joe, a human being who loves life. The
one in greatest need gives life to science. And the heart of
pity gives science to life.

CHAPTER 10

FLORENCE NIGHTINGALE: ONE BY THE OTHER

I had rather feel compunction,
than understand the definition thereof.

—Thomas à Kempis

On *Florence Nightingale* and *Notes on Nursing*: The Nurse Speaks

Heidegger finds in being there (G. *da-sein*, there-being) the essence of human being. Care is the *being* of being there. We are the *there* of being there, the place and time where the being of care is revealed through our silence, our speech, our actions.[1] What is it like to choose to be there in a situation of illness; to be there, a nurse? Florence Nightingale (1820-1910) chose to be there, a nurse, in the Crimean War and to fight for the rest of her life for adequate medical care for British soldiers. Excerpts from her biography by Woodham-Smith, "the small, still beginning, the simple hardship, the silent and, gradual struggle upwards," give life to her instructions to student nurses.[2]

What Nursing Does

i. *Memories in action, or Learning from experience.*
ii. *Nursing helps nature heal.*

i. (1897) The relics, the representations of the Crimean War! What are they? They are first the tremendous lessons we had to learn from its tremendous blunders and ignorances.

143

And next they are Trained Nurses and the progress of Hygiene. These are the "representations" of the Crimean War. (p. 425)

ii. Pathology teaches the harm that disease has done. But it teaches nothing more. We know nothing of the principle of health the positive of which pathology is the negative, except from observation and experience. And nothing but observation and experience will teach us the ways to maintain or bring back the state of health. It is often thought that medicine is the curative process. It is no such thing; medicine is the surgery of functions, as surgery proper is that of limbs and organs. Neither can cure, nature alone cures. Surgery removes the bullet out of the limb, which is an obstruction to cure, but nature heals the wound. So it is with medicine; the function of an organ becomes obstructed; medicine, so far as we know, assists nature to remove the obstruction, but does nothing more. And what nursing has to do in either case, is to put the patient in the best condition for nature to act upon him. (p. 110)

"Nursing still does that," the nurse says.[3] The patient is taught the benefit of and procedures for preventative measures, such as hygiene and inoculation, as well as general health care in response to the disease process, such as diet, rest and exercise. But nursing must also respond to the requirements of increased technology. With dialysis, the process of nature is stopped. With transplantation, the process of nature is reversed. The fulfillment of this paradox is a healthy dialysis person or a healthy transplant person. This intervention into the process of nature requires refined techniques, which in turn require more questions to be asked to ascertain the patient's condition. The nurse speaks a technical vocabulary concerning the disease process, tests and treatment which she explains to the patient in terms of the purpose of the procedure and what the experience will be like.

Ruth[4] couldn't sleep. She was demanding, grouchy, and nagging. As she began to listen to the nurse's description of her experience in terms of a disease process that many people undergo, the fear of the unknown became a pathway to follow. She began to understand this difficult time as a time for choosing among limited alternatives for a healthful way of living (choosing to follow a restrictive diet, for example). She became aware that she could choose her attitude in all this. She chose kindness, courtesy, consideration.

The nurse cannot change the progression of the disease, but she can help to ease the experience. She can be there, a nurse.

Seeing Illness

Being with the patient is the "praxis" of observation.[5]

Nursing has to nurse living bodies and spirits. (p. 412)

The most important practical lesson that can be given to nurses is to teach them what to observe—how to observe—what symptoms indicate medical improvement—what the reverse—which are of importance—which are of none—which are the evidence of neglect—and of what kind of neglect. (p. 88)

The initial months of nurses' training are designed to teach the nursing student to 'see' particular indicators of disease. For example, pallor, swelling, and uremic odor are indicators of kidney disease. But the nurse learns to 'see' the effect of these indicators in the lives of her patients through many experiences. While observational data and skills are first taught and then practised, the teaching of experience begins with the sense that "something is not right," says the nurse, and slowly becomes articulate. The meaning of the indicators of disease in the patient's life is pain.

The nurse sees shallowness around the eyes, greyness in the skin, a grimace when a painful area is touched, lethargy which can be due to the pain of movement, listlessness from the supreme effort to undergo pain. She misses seeing the accustomed gestures, the light in the eyes. In the missing, there is the hope for the return. Can the patient come through the pain? The nurse's presence is the embodiment of that hope.

Light at Night

Night care: night rounds; night provisions.

> One of the nurses described accompanying her on her night
> rounds. 'It seemed an endless walk. As we slowly passed
> along the silence was profound; very seldom did a moan
> or a cry from those deeply suffering fall on our ear. A dim
> light burned here and there. Miss Nightingale carried her
> lantern which she would set down before she bent over any
> of her patients. I much admired her manner to the men—
> it was so tender and kind.' (p. 160)

> A good nurse will always make sure that no door or window
> in her patient's room shall rattle or creak; that no blind
> or curtain shall, by any change of wind through the open
> window, be made to flap—especially will she be careful of
> all this before she leaves her patients for the night. If you
> wait till your patients tell you or remind you of these things,
> where is the use of their having a nurse? There are more
> shy than exacting patients, in all classes, and many a
> patient passes a bad night, time after time, rather than
> remind his nurse every night of all the things she has
> forgotten. (p. 36)

"It's the little things that count," the nurse says. When
giving out medications in the evening, she asks the patient
about his or her preference for night care. "A glass of water
by the bedside? A light in the room? Shades drawn? Untuck
toes? Another blanket?"

Lights dimmed and curtains drawn have a quieting effect
for one patient while, for another, bright light is cheering.

> When John[6] was dying, he wanted to see things, see people
> pass by. His wife left at 10:00 P.M. after a twelve hour vigil
> and the light was his contact with life when she was gone.
> He waited through the night for the day, the return of his
> beloved visitor.

The depth of time in the quiet of the night is accentuated
or alleviated by the light, the noise of the intercom, the tones

of conversation, the sound of footsteps, the nurse come in for night care or to check for night symptoms, such as restlessness and need for oxygen which can increase in intensity because of anxiety over wakefulness. The hours between 2:00 and 4:00 A.M. are the "longest." The patient awake during these hours often tells the morning nurse, "The night was very long." So the patient waits for sleep and for the morning, perhaps for sleep in the morning. The nurse waits for the morning and for the sleep she needs after a night of work.

Bright light is not sufficient to return us to the day. Day is heralded by the hospital clatter. The patient hears time pass with the food wagons, the intercom now in competition with conversation and laughter, the routines. And the patient watches time pass, the nurse's quick gestures and pace, the cleaning staff's activity, and the doctor's rounds. Time skims along the surface of the bustling day and shelters the patient and nurse in its passing.

Perhaps watching and hearing time pass helped John recall his time, the nurse says. "I've had a good life. I've raised my children. I've done what I wanted." Time that has passed stands still like the stillness of the wakeful night. Time that has passed becomes a song, and the refrain is sung over and over by those who remember, "He had a good life." Good memories are a light at night for the patient, nurse, and family and friends.

The Presence of Care

The honesty of silence; and of speech.

> When such a one [a wounded soldier] looked and saw that the honored Lady in Chief was patiently standing beside him—and with lips closely set and hands folded—decreeing herself to go through the pain of witnessing pain, he used to fall into the mood of obeying her silent command and—finding strange support in her presence—bring himself to submit and endure. (p. 160)
>
> What a convenience it would be if there were any single person to whom he [the patient] could speak simply and

> openly without pulling the string upon himself of this
> shower-bath of silly hopes and encouragements; to whom
> he could express his wishes and directions without that
> person persisting in saying 'I hope that it will please God
> yet to give you twenty years' or, 'You have a long life of
> activity before you.' (p. 86)

The nurse and the patient must trust that each other is
trying to help. The nurse can speak about a "compliant" or
a "noncompliant" patient. The patient can speak about a
"judge" or an "empathizer."⁷ But the attitude of trust which
binds the nurse and patient in a common endeavor finds
expression through the experience of the family. "If my father,
my mother, my son were here, how would I want them to be
treated? How would I want to be treated?" the nurse asks.
And so, the medical significance of the procedure dwells as
surely in the presence of care as it does in the promise of
medical theory and practise. Paradoxically, the nurse is
strengthened to carry out painful procedures by her commitment to the patient *as if* she were a family member. This care,
she in turn must give over to other professionals when
members of her own family are ill—her senses dulled with
her own pain, she could not carry out her nursing responsibilities. The abiding *as if* is a condition for nursing care.
Yet, this *as if* does not automatically establish trust
between the nurse and the patient. "How it comes about, I'm
not sure," says the nurse. But she recognizes trust in silence,
and in speech, even in the tone of speech.

> Sometimes silence is a comfort. You don't have to say things
> to fill the silence. Sometimes just sitting by a patient's bed,
> holding a hand—there is a lot of comfort in that which you
> cannot speak. Bring in a hot water bottle without being
> asked, pull the blind. Just a feeling of trust.

Other gestures shared in silence 'speak' trust—the
invitation of a smile or outstretched hand, a reassuring pat,
a wink, a wave. But the nurse speaks of the other silence,
too, the silence where these gestures are witheld or ignored,
the silence that needs speech.

> Another nurse and I went in to see a young man who was
> distressed about his disease process. The curtains were
> drawn around his bed with the light over the bed off. Also,
> he didn't have the light on in the room. He had his T.V. set
> plugged in. We couldn't get a "yes" or "no" answer out of
> him. We asked him how he felt about his kidney disease.
> He took a long time, he didn't tell us quickly... The next
> night we went in, the curtains were open and the lights
> were on in the room but not over the bed. We talked a bit
> more...

In this situation, speech was the purveyor of trust. The
nurse continues, "Sometimes, people who go into themselves
don't really wish to be alone, they just don't know how to
approach you about how they are feeling." This young man
spoke out of a history of misfortune. He had lost his job and
now, his health. How would he provide for his wife and small
child? His home was already a place of homelessness.
Technology could not answer for it. But a nurse was there.
Was the nurse there in spite of the technology of medical care?
In addition to that technology? With that technology? In other
ways? In the examples cited are the questions that ask for
deeper understanding. What does it mean to be there, a nurse?

To Be There, a Nurse

To Be There, a Nurse, is to Ease the Dis-ease of Illness

From one day to the next, the nurse participates in and
often initiates the small changes which aid recovery. When
the patient is lost in the complexity of previously simple tasks
such as washing, dressing, eating, the nurse is there, doing
for and with the patient what the patient cannot do. During
such encounters, the nurse 'establishes rapport' with the
patient. But the expression 'establishes rapport' belies the
artfulness and skill of the nurse who helps a patient stand
the second day after major surgery. The patient must will
to stand with the nurse against the pain. The nurse sponsors
a mutual endeavor, a mutual accomplishment.

To Be There, a Nurse, is to Remember that the Ill Person Feels Far From Home

Whether for diagnosis or treatment medical technology is formidable. The patient may feel like the junction of tubes and wires, the extension of a machine or even the target of a machine. Barbara Coleman describes her experience of cobalt treatments following brain surgery for a malignant tumor.

> The first time I took it the radiologist laid it on the line for me. He said, "You will go into a room with concrete walls and you will be bald for the rest of your life." I went into that concrete room. I was alone. Everything is operated by remote control. They transmit orders to you through an intercom. It was depersonalization at its zenith.[8]

Perhaps the radiation would kill only the cancer cells and the hair cells. What of the mind, the will, the emotions? The technology of medical care asks us, "Is life that precious?"

The technology of medical care must become routine for the nurse to carry out duties effectively. But the nurse must remember that the homeland of the heart gives meaning to technological care. The patient suffers technological care for the sake of the homeland of the heart. The language of the heart is the simple sharing of anecdotes and news about family and friends, work, recreation, and worship. The nurse who is mindful of the homeland speaks the language of the heart.

To Be There, a Nurse, is to See Pain in the Light of Hope

Hope is the nurse's promise of help, asserted in the greeting, "Good morning, I am your nurse today." Hope is the nurse's assurance that post-operative pain will pass. And hope is the nurse's presence when pain does not pass. Elizabeth Lord, a nurse who recovered from cancer, describes her relationship with Jean, who was dying of cancer. The light of hope she gave was not the promise of recovery but the presence of care. She gave of herself.

Jean has been here three weeks and now as I walk into her room, we don't say much . . .
She received the last rites of the church a week ago and tells me so. We have talked about God and how to pray and why God has permitted this to happen. It is no longer simply a nurse-patient relationship; it is much more. She depends on me for reassurance, understanding, compassion, and, yes, even love.[9]

Has the nurse gone beyond what nursing is? What of the emotional stress, and the nurse's other responsibilities in hospital and at home? Has the nurse found what nursing is? What of these last days of life in a hospital room, and the earth and sky are beautiful, and memories glow with the warmth of life, and pain is everywhere? Will the nurse who gives of herself find herself emptied or strengthened?

I see her body lose its tension; she smiles and thanks me, says I have made her feel better, more relaxed about everything.[10]

A little kindness and compassion, and the face of pain relaxes for a moment in a smile; the voice from death whispers, "Thank you." A little kindness, a little compassion— a little light in the shadow of pain and death. And this light shines on the nurse, too. She receives the smile, the deep gratitude; she experiences wonder at the patient's courage and dignity. She gives from the heart and receives to the heart. Yes, also the grief. Where is the light in grief?

CHAPTER 11

LORD TENNYSON: ONE WITHOUT THE OTHER

You will always miss me,
but that does not mean
missing out on life.

—Pauline Erickson

On "In Memoriam": The Mother Speaks

Tennyson wrote "In Memoriam, A. H. H."[1] as a tribute to Arthur Henry Hallam, his closest friend who died at sea. The poem journeys through the experience of grief, the one without the other, from the early confusion, to acceptance, to peace, and even joy. First published in 1850, the poem led Queen Victoria to offer Tennyson the laureateship.

To Speak About Grief

Language fails to express grief.

> I sometimes hold it half a sin
> To put in words the grief I feel;
> For words, like Nature, half reveal
> And half conceal the soul within.

The "sorrow of language" writes Merleau-Ponty, is that words cannot express all we want to say. How can we convey our grief? Language lives; there are no words for death. And words do not mean the same to everyone. "Experiences of grief vary to such an extent that intended and interpreted meanings may be diametrically opposed," Mother writes.[2] For example, "It's all for the best," may sound callous though it is well meant. So we venture, "We're sorry... Is there anything we can do to help?" We respond, "You have done so much already." And we give and receive flowers or fruit, or a handshake, or a hug. We give ourselves in these conventional gestures. But we stay ourselves in these conventional gestures, too. We do not want to hurt those we meant to help.

Can language alleviate grief?

> But, for the unquiet heart and brain
> A use in measured language lies;
> The sad mechanic exercise,
> Like dull narcotics, numbing pain.

We ponder the events that happened before death as if we could change the outcome. 'If only we had... How could we have... Perhaps we should have...' Late into the night we talk and in the morning, we rise with the same thoughts. Death is with us in the morning. We could not talk it through.

Language shelters grief.

> In words, like weeds, I'll wrap me o'er,
> Like coarsest clothes against the cold;
> But that large grief which these enfold
> Is given in outline and no more. (p. 122)

We wrap ourselves in words to protect us from the bitter cold of the grief in our soul. To grief belongs the silence of our life, the silence of days lived with the one who is gone. That great bulk of silent time is now a mist. Language begins to penetrate the mist: language is the path to "the Soul within." Language is also the path to the world outside. Mother writes, "We share grief with a devoted friend: this expression of grief in words and tears, gives release to the pain and anguish dwelling in the depths of our being." Love is giving of ourselves in cards and notes and letters.

Gradually, thoughts turn from death to life. Recollections take on new meaning as treasures gathered from a way of living that have the name of the one we love. Gradually, too, the routines of daily life enfold us as we listen to friends chat about family, work, and weather. The language of friendship shelters our grief as we return to the workaday world.

Dark House

The house is the last vestige of friendship.

> Dark house, by which once more I stand
> Here in the long unlovely street,
> Doors, where my heart was used to beat
> So quickly, waiting for a hand,
>
> A hand that can be clasp'd no more
> Behold me, for I cannot sleep,
> And like a guilty thing I creep
> At earliest morning to the door.

We go to the place of our memory but the house is dark. It was the hand of our friend that invited us into the house. But the hand of friendship is gone: in Mother's words, "a treasured home; a barren house." The Old Norse word for "home" is *heimr*, 'residence, world.'[3] Once this home embraced us in its world: we belonged here; but the "house"—Old English, *hús*, 'shelter'—cannot shelter us from death.[4] The house stands empty for us. There is no one watching at the window, no one waiting at the door. No rush of greetings and silence and sudden laughter. Mother knows, "All that remain are silent photographs on the mantel."

Bleakness engulfs us.

> He is not here; but far away
> The noise of life begins again,
> And ghastly thro' the drizzling rain
> On the bald street breaks the blank day. (p. 124)

Mother writes, "The cold harsh fact is that life goes on in the world as though nothing changed in our own private world." There is a notice in the newspaper. A gathering of friends. A service in the church. We resume our workaday responsibilities. But we are estranged from the purposeful rhythm of daily life. Traffic lights blink red and green and people stop and go. The people stop and go. We have no-where to go; no reason to stop or go.

The Paradox of Calm

The silence of calm

> Calm is the morn without a sound,
> Calm as to suit a calmer grief,
> And only thro' the faded leaf
> The chestnut pattering to the ground;

The light of calm

> Calm and still light on yon great plain
> That sweeps with all its autumn bowers,
> And crowded farms and lessening towers,
> To mingle with the bounding main;

The air of calm

> Calm and deep peace in this wide air,
> These leaves that redden to the fall,
> And in my heart, if calm at all
> If any calm, a calm despair;

The rest of calm

> Calm on the seas, and silver sleep,
> And waves that sway themselves in rest,
> And dead calm in that noble breast
> Which heaves but with the heaving deep. (p.127)

Exhausted from the wild grief of the first days and nights, we wake to "still light," "deep peace," "and waves that sway themselves in rest." "All the qualities of calm in nature penetrate the entire human being. In nature, we find solace and companionship," writes Mother. Standing thus in nature, we can yet stand apart from nature when we ponder life and death, responding to the silence, light, air, and rest of calm with "calm despair" because of a "dead calm." "But is this a true 'calm'? Is there not always hope and faith as in living with the memory of love? Can someone who was loved and needed ever really leave our lives?"[5]

Sharing a Life

Sharing burdens:

> I know that this was Life,—the track
> Whereon with equal feet we fared;
> And then, as now, the day prepared
> The daily burden for the back.

you needed me;

> But this it was that made me move
> As light as carrier-birds in air;
> I loved the weight I had to bear,
> Because it needed help of Love;

I needed you.

> Nor could I weary, heart or limb,
> When mighty Love would cleave in twain
> The lading of a single pain,
> And part it, giving half to him. (p. 137)

The treasure of the days that are gone dwells, not in the ease of the days, but in the responsible work of the days, a work of love, shared in love, lightened by love. "During World War II," writes Mother, "a poster commonly seen was that of a boy carrying a sickly younger boy. Above was the caption, 'He's not heavy, Mister. He's my brother.' Love carried the burden. In the same way, big sister helps little sister, as when our daughter carried her younger sister up the school stairs on her back after the other children were in class because of the bone pain the younger one suffered. That was the last time she was at school. It is always easier to be the one who can help than the one who needs help."

Immortal treasure

> I hold it true, whate'er befall;
> I feel it, when I sorrow most;
> 'Tis better to have loved and lost
> Than never to have loved at all. (p. 138)

"To pass through life uncaring would be mere existence. To give love to a fellow being is to reflect the image of God," Mother writes. Through the eyes of love, we see with William Blake, "the world in a grain of sand and eternity in an hour." The hour, like the grain of sand, holds the possibility of the universe. The possibility of the universe is meaningful to us as the possibility for the one we love. Our possibility blossoms when love constrains us to live for the other. Death does not end our cherished responsibility to live for the other.

> If ye break faith with us who die
> We shall not sleep. . .[6]

The life we shared is never lost though never found again.

Life Stops (The First Christmas After)

We are apprehensive;

> With trembling fingers did we weave
> The holly round the Christmas hearth;
> A rainy cloud possess'd the earth,
> And sadly fell our Christmas-eve.

we pretend to be glad.

At our old pastimes in the hall
We gamboll'd, making vain pretence
Of gladness, with an awful sense
Of one mute Shadow watching all.

Our circle is smaller.

We paused: the winds were in the beech;
We heard them sweep the winter land;
And in a circle hand-in-hand
Sat silent, looking each at each.

The present seems to echo the past, it has no voice of its own.

Then echo-like our voices rang;
We sung, tho' every eye was dim,
A merry song we sang with him
Last year; impetuously we sang.

We speak our loss:

We ceased; a gentler feeling crept
Upon us: surely rest is meet.
"They rest," we said, "their sleep is sweet,"
And silence follow'd, and we wept.

we speak our hope.

Our voices took a higher range;
Once more we sang: "They do not die
Nor lose their mortal sympathy,
Nor change to us, although they change;

Rise, happy morn, rise, holy morn,
Draw forth the cheerful day from night:
O Father, touch the east, and light
The light that shone when hope was born. (pp. 139,140)

Christmas is celebrated as if it were the same Christmas as last year and the year before. But we cannot hide from our grief. Wherever we look, a treasured smile is missing. Whenever we speak, a treasured voice is gone. "With dismay," Mother writes, "we cast a backward glance down the corridor of time. Our hope that the magic of Christmas could return to us our human treasures is a fleeting hope for a fleeting season." Yet the Christmas celebration survives the loss of ones so greatly missed: a child was born in Bethlehem. "Hope is born at Christmas, and we move with a lighter step and new resolve into the unknown future."

"Be Near Me"

Physical signs of death

> Be near me when my light is low,
> When the blood creeps, and the nerves prick
> And tingle, and the heart is sick,
> And all the wheels of being slow.

We sit beside the one we love, alert to the rhythm of breathing, the slightest movement, a momentary frown. We sit so near, yet so far away. We say over and over, "Where there is life, there is hope." We look for life. We wait for death.

Emotional signs of death

> Be near me when the sensuous frame
> Is rack'd with pangs that conquer trust;
> And Time, a maniac scattering dust,
> And Life, a Fury slinging flame.

Death takes time, and time is a "maniac." There is a moment that takes an hour, an hour that lasts a day, a day that is unending night. The clock no longer orders our life. We eat lunch at midnight if we remember to eat at all. We stay where we are needed, and we need to stay.

Spiritual signs of death

> Be near me when my faith is dry,
> And me the flies of latter spring,
> That lay their eggs, and sting and sing
> And weave their petty cells and die.

What is the sum of our days? Even if we look, not to the vastness of eternity, but to the vastness of history, our life is nothing. Our life has meaning in this moment—always just past, always new—this moment that calls us to respond, like Martin Luther, "Here I stand. I cannot do otherwise."

The need for companionship

> Be near me when I fade away,
> To point the term of human strife,
> And on the low dark verge of life
> The twilight of eternal day. (pp. 152, 153)

Mother writes, "One of life's greatest sorrows is that of loneliness, reinforced by the plight of helplessness, as the beloved body of the one we love fails to function normally." In the loneliness of our grief, we remember death. Our "heart is sick," we are "rack'd with pangs," our "faith is dry." Our soul "cries out for the companionship of its Maker and for the nearness of loved ones," writes Mother. "Be near me. . ."

Learning to Trust

Can what is evil or aimless yield good?

> O, yet we trust that somehow good
> Will be the final goal of ill,
> To pangs of nature, sins of will,
> Deflects of doubt, and taints of blood;
>
> That nothing walks with aimless feet;
> That not one life shall be destroy'd,
> Or cast as rubbish to the void,
> When God hath made the pile complete;

Is the end of knowledge the beginning of trust?

> Behold, we know not anything;
> I can but trust that good shall fall
> At last—far off—at last, to all,
> And every winter change to spring.

> So runs my dream; but what am I?
> An infant crying in the night;
> An infant crying for the light,
> And with no language but a cry. (p. 155)

What does 'trust' mean? The Old English word for trust, *tréowian*, means 'to believe'; Old Norse, *traust*, means 'confidence'; Old High German, *tróst*, means 'fidelity.'[7] With confidence, we believe God is faithful: we trust. God is faithful. Mother writes, "As we trust that every winter will change to spring, so we trust that the seasons of our human existence will change from faltering hope to vigorous new life. Yet hope wanes through times of waiting and enduring. Our perplexity so often ends in a cry: 'what is man that thou art mindful of him and the son of man that thou visitest him?'[8] We want to know life's purpose when so much we experience works at cross-purpose to the good." We know that day is the other side of night. We cannot come to fully know. We can come to fully trust.

To be Silent About Grief

Expressing praise is a vain show of grief.

> I care not in these fading days
> To raise a cry that lasts not long,
> And round thee with the breeze of song
> To stir a little dust of praise.

The meaning of his life is in what he set out to do.

> Thy leaf has perish'd in the green
> And, while we breathe beneath the sun,

The world which credits what is done
Is cold to all that might have been.

His greatness cannot be measured here.

So here shall silence guard thy fame;
But somewhere, out of human view,
Whate'er thy hands are set to do
Is wrought with tumult of acclaim. (p. 168)

The one we love is wrapped in silence as we are wrapped in words. We ponder what he gave, what he would have given in time. We would praise him if words could express our debt of love and gratitude to him for being all he could be. "Words cannot re-create him. Therefore, our silence, more eloquent than words, 'speaks' our loss," writes Mother. Silence shines: silence shrouds. Silence is the voice of the dead.

Life Goes On (The Second Christmas After)

We live through grief.

Who show'd a token of distress?
No single tear, no mark of pain
O sorrow, then can sorrow wane?
O grief, can grief be changed to less?

Grief marks our soul, not our face.

O last regret, regret can die!
No—mixt with all this mystic frame,
Her deep relations are the same,
But with long use her tears are dry. (p. 170)

Life appears to win over death. Mother writes, "Tears do not visibly flow. There are inward tears." And softly spoken or gently thought, 'Here he opened the gift I gave him'; 'There she sang the Christmas songs.' Other Christmases come so close. We cannot say how close the tears. For grief is not less than last Christmas. But the memories are gentler now, more "softly outlined."

Eulogy

Song of Faith

> Perplext in faith, but pure in deeds,
> At last he beat his music out.
> There lives more faith in honest doubt,
> Believe me, than in half the creeds.

strong doubt;

> He fought his doubts and gather'd strength,
> He would not make his judgment blind,
> He faced the spectres of the mind
> And laid them; thus he came at length

strong faith;

> To find a stronger faith his own,
> And Power was with him in the night,
> Which makes the darkness and the light,
> And dwells not in the light alone,

strong commitment.

> But in the darkness and the cloud,
> As over Sinai's peaks of old,
> While Israel made their gods of gold,
> Altho' the trumpet blew so loud. (p. 189)

Words cannot express our debt of love and gratitude; yet, here, a eulogy, not to praise the end of his work, but to ponder the beginning. We must try to tell the meanings of a life so dear. He believed through doubt. Mother writes, "The battles with doubt are part of the clarifying process in making harmony out of discord. The struggles endow strength and a clearer, stronger, truer faith, a faith that heeds the clarion call of the trumpet."

Song of Hope

Ring out, wild bells, to the wild sky,
The flying cloud, the frosty light:
The year is dying in the night;
Ring out, wild bells, and let him die.

Ring out the old, ring in the new,
Ring, happy bells, across the snow:
The year is going, let him go;
Ring out the false, ring in the true.

Ring out the grief that saps the mind,
For those that here we see no more;
Ring out the feud of rich and poor,
Ring in redress to all mankind.

Ring out a slowly dying cause,
And ancient forms of party strife;
Ring in the nobler modes of life,
With sweeter manners, purer laws.

Ring out the want, the care, the sin,
The faithless coldness of the times;
Ring out, ring out my mournful rhymes,
But ring the fuller minstrel in.

Ring out false pride in place and blood,
The civic slander and the spite;
Ring in the love of truth and right,
Ring in the common love of good.

Ring out old shapes of foul disease;
Ring out the narrowing lust for gold;
Ring out the thousand wars of old,
Ring in the thousand years of peace.

Ring in the valiant man and free,
The larger heart, the kindlier hand;
Ring out the darkness of the land,
Ring in the Christ that is to be. (pp. 198, 199)

"Ring out, wild bells." The Old Year takes with it its own darkness. "We anticipate the New Year with a buoyant joy," Mother writes, and she thinks of these Bible verses: "I shall go to him, but he shall not return to me" and "I know that my Redeemer lives."⁹ And wild as our grief the wild bells ring! Strong as our hope the strong clappers strike! Free as the wind the free notes chime! Our grieving never ends: our hope is strong again: our love is freely bound. Wild and strong and free!

CHAPTER 12

THE HOMECOMING

The Master is come, and calleth for thee.

—John 11:28

Children of God

Is there a name for logos? A Person to whom we can turn when we begin a journey like Abraham? A Person who will give us faith and teach us to live in faith? A Person whose presence will transform the sacrifice into a blessing of hope and joy and peace? Name of logos—Word of God, Jesus.[1] I give my life to You in this hour also.

A boy who had cerebral palsy attended Bible Camp where the other boys mimicked his movement, his speech. Each evening, one cabin was responsible for devotions for the entire assembly. The boys in his cabin chose him. He came, speaking haltingly, his words breaking under the awesome silence of each sacred breath, "I love Jesus and Jesus loves me." The assembly was silent. He had spoken, "not like the stranger or the guest, but like the child at home." How can we ever hope unless we can always hope? I look to the manger, the cross and the empty tomb. My hope in illness and death is the comfort of my Creator's eternal love, embodied in the life of Jesus and in the lives of you who care. Let God make us in the image of His Son. This is our "sacrifice of praise."[2] And in the weariness and rigor of illness, we will learn to rest our souls like a child at home. We are "children of God."[3]

Eddie's Homecoming

When my oldest brother Eddie died, my mother wrote of his life in "The Shepherd," the Canadian Lutheran periodical at that time: Edward Theodore James Olson, son of Pastor and Mrs. H. O. Olson of Moose Jaw, Saskatchewan, was born on June 27, 1949. He was granted entrance to his heavenly home on September 10, 1959.

In spite of recurring illness and frequent hospitalization all his days, Eddie lived a normal life. By nature he was energetic. God-given grace enabled him to remain constantly patient and contagiously optimistic. Blessed with an active and inquiring mind, days or months abed at home or in the hospital were spent contructively; and being an avid reader, he readily maintained his grades at school. He progressed in music and for a time participated in the junior choir.

Eddie's life became a ministry at home. When collapse of both kidneys finally confined him to a wheelchair and then to bed, he spoke of himself as committed to God in the way His Maker saw best. He talked readily about Jesus, his Saviour, his beautiful homeland where there would be no sickness, and of the glorious day of resurrection. As his days on earth drew to a close, his faith blossomed so that during intense suffering he consoled those at his bedside who loved him the most. On the morning of his departure he expressed the desire that God would soon take him unto Himself in Heaven. "And now our hearts, wiser than eyes, can see him there."

Thus, by the hand of a child, we are led to nobler heights to view the grandeur of God's might, to experience His matchless love, and perceive that His wisdom is infinite.

> "Looking ever upward we can say:
> Thy day has come, not gone;
> Thy sun has risen, not set;
> Thy life is now beyond
> The reach of death or change,
> Not ended—but begun."

CHAPTER 13

EPILOGUE

> My heart wants to reach out to you
> and to ask you to be strong. . .
>
> —T. T. Aoki

Student of a Research Question

I am a student of the research question that characterizes hermeneutic phenomenology, "What is life like?" This research question fills me with its urgency because it dwells in my life and asks me how I ought to live. I study, not to master the research question, but to live in it with understanding. Paradoxically, in my search to understand the research question, I must step away from it. My step away from the research question is reflection, not reflection that would build a structure for life, but reflection that would search for the structures—themes of life and give these themes a home in written language and in the lives of the readers. What has it been like to learn to reflect—read, interview, write—phenomenologically?

1. Lived Experience Questions Us.

Recollection of 1971. I was waiting in the dimly-lit hall of the dialysis unit. I saw Jim[1] leaning against the wall, gasping for air. He was hunchbacked and barrelchested with bone disease. I could see the pain vibrating in him, burning him. And darkly, the fatigue encircled his eyes. Staring at him, I feared my pain.

Then he smiled at me. And in his eyes, I saw how strong, this suffering man; how strong, his kindness towards me, how strong, his dignity. I believed if he could live, so could I. I came away from the encounter with new courage.

2. Illumination of Experience by Reading.

The learning I lived in that encounter was wordless until I read *Man's Search for Meaning* by Victor Frankl a decade later. Frankl writes that suffering requires a choice between futures—hidden futures since any way of life appears to be death to the onlooker.

> Everything can be taken from a man but one thing: the last of human freedoms—to choose one's attitude in any given set of circumstances, to choose one's own way.[2]

3. Understanding Lived Experience.

Understanding the experience (1) was partly evoked by reading the excerpt (2). Dialogue with the text is interpretation. The interpretation is always one possible interpretation, the one that fulfills my need.

4. Emergence of a Theme.

As theorist, I am also witness to the meaning of my interpretation by the way I live in the question. The literary excerpt and my response to it do not encapsulate my learning, closing the matter once and for all. These statements are my question because they question me. There is a mystery here, a miracle: I knew a man who chose to suffer well. And there is a community of shared meaning here, a theme: We can choose to suffer well.

But what is the light by which such a choice comes to life in the life of an individual? What is this humiliation of the will that enables one to live in humility? What is this "healing process" whereby "one can actually improve even as the body disintegrates?"[3] ask medical sociologists, Bergsma and Thomasa.

5. *Return to Lived Experience.*

These questions resonating in the theme draw us back into the research question. To be drawn back into the research question is to be impelled forward into life to participate in the mystery and the miracle expressed in the theme.

Interview with a dialysis nurse, September 1984: "Mike made a deep impression on me.[4] He was a triple amputee on dialysis because of diabetes. He was always cheering *you* up. He did all sorts of marvelous things—he worked with a physiotherapist to develop films to help new amputees, he invited nurses and patients into his home." The nurse expressed the theme of her encounters with Mike: "We can choose to live to the very fullest of our capabilities, working to discover our full potential."

The theme, "We can choose to suffer well," is made visible as an action by this related theme. What is the essence of this action—Mike's cheerfulness, Jim's smile? Is it not hospitality in the Greek sense? But Mike and Jim were the strangers. . .

6. *Once Again, The Journey.*

Once again, we stand at the threshold of the beginning. Once again, we "cast [our] bread upon the waters" in expectation of the promise, "You will find it after many days."[5] Once again, this tension of casting away and finding is expressed in the question and the theme; the theme in the question and the question in the theme, and the journey between.

Researching Phenomenological Texts

As a student of a research question that is conditioned by my coming to ask it out of my life of dialysis, I have been commited to search for understanding in texts that are authored in a strong way. As in learning to speak a foreign language, I had to learn to think from the inside of the authors' textual expressions. I could not stop reading at points of difficulty. Also, since the enigmatic phrase dwells within the wholeness of the authors' work, I needed to continue to read. There is beauty in the enigmatic phrase, the glimmer of meaning, the recognition, "I have not thought this thought before." I want to understand! As I continued to read and reflect, the enigmatic phrase became the apex of simplicity and clarity. I found life there and I sought to welcome the phrase and surround it with the writing that reflection upon it had sponsored. The phrase now spoke from within my writing; it belonged to my thought about the research question.

There is also the phrase that jumps out from the text, laden with meaning. I received such a phrase as a discovery. It is the clear articulation of a thought that was not ready to be written, inspiration for my writing.

The indented style of the longer quotation was meant to help show its meaning. Not only do I defer to the author's way of writing but I recognize life through the author's unique expression, and the life cannot be separated from the words. Also, I wanted to be understood as I had understood the quotation because I have my own words, too: the quotation is part of my research biography, part of my tradition as a student of the research question, "What is life like?"

Yields of the Literary Texts

The literary excerpts were received like a gift from the literary authors, words from life that gave me insight into the life of illness. The authors stood within life to ask, "What is life?" through their writing of the life of one in community. The deep questioning of the uniqueness of the individual in community, love for the other personified, was a pathway for the research question, "What is life like?"

I searched for the words that enabled these authors— researchers of life, to write life. So I tried to speak with persons who shared my search for understanding, persons who speak with the wisdom that dedication to the other teaches.

As interviewers, in the phenomenological tradition, we do not come with questions. Our coming is a question. Our attitude is openness: each interview is different from the other, each person is unique. Yet my participation was guided

by the expression of life in the literary text. The style of
research writing was subject to the manner in which life was
articulated through the interview in response to the literary
text. For example, in "Ivan Ilyitch: One against the Other
Searches for the Other," the death of Ivan Ilyitch 'speaks' as
a parable of life in a technological society. The quality of
parable was heightened by the chaplain's message of mercy
in response to the excerpts from *The Death of Ivan Ilyitch* and
abides in the chapter as a sustained reference to Ivan, Vanya,
he: Ivan Ilyitch is the example.

However, in "Doctor Rieux: One for the Other," I wrote
as the doctor spoke, not of Doctor Rieux's life in *The Plague*,
but of the doctor's response to his life, a comparison of thought
and action in similar and differing medical situations. So the
medical situation is the example.

In "Florence Nightingale: One by the Other," the nurse
responded to generalizations concerning nursing care that
came from the heart of Miss Nightingale's experiences with
wounded soldiers. Through the nurse's examples of her
experiences of nursing care, she has brought these generalizations back to life.

In "Pauline Ericson: One with the Other," the responses
to excerpts from Pauline's diary were the articulation of the
meanings of my experiences of illness in a family where my
brothers and sisters also had kidney failure. It is the writing
of the years we shared, the love we shared, the we of illness.

In "Lord Tennyson: One without the Other," my mother
and I found it difficult to speak our grief, our response to "In
Memoriam, A. H. H." This poem questions and cares for our
silence in grief, the silence of the creature before the Creator.
This silence belongs to the written word. Mother's written
responses to the excerpts keep this quality of silence. We had
few words for grief, and we could find no more.

Yields of the Writing

The other chapters asked for more words, for the further
articulation of the central themes. First, I tried to journey
with those who had experienced illness as Kierkegaard

journeyed with Abraham in his writing. Then, I tried to respond to each journey thematically as Kierkegaard had responded to Abraham's journey with his expression of themes of faith. The action of journeying was thematized in the central thematic expressions, "Letting Go of the Things" and "The Struggle to Be Born into a Life of Illness." Illness is an individual journey and the themes of illness became the themes of personal change in light of what never changes: logos. Reflection at the end of the journey was highlighted in the central thematic expressions, "The Heart of Pity" and "To Be There, a Nurse." Illness is a journey to the beginning of community and the themes of illness became the themes of a way of being in light of what never changes: logos.

The themes have been the strength of my journeys as a student of the research question, "What is life like?" But each journey has been a different history, so the way of expressing the themes for each journey has been different—yet there is unity to the thematic content. For example, when a journey of illness started with the question, "Why ought Ivan die?", the thematic expressions were different than a journey that started with the question, "How is self-pity honorable?" However, these questions demonstrated a showing power in the lives of Ivan and Pauline as they lived through the questions to the place of rest. Such questions were given to me for research, questions that are always too difficult. How could anyone articulate the showing power?

All the work of phenomenological research is for the writing, and the writing is the most difficult work of all. The writing is the research rather than the report of research. For example, when I am alone, pen in hand and paper, there are no words unless I write them; there is no silence unless the words I write keep the silence. The writing is a way of reflection.

Phenomenological research writing is autobiographical in the sense that I want to understand more deeply what I have experienced so I can love life better. Writing my experience helps me reflect, reflecting on my experience helps me write. But because I reflect on my experience in dialogue with the thematic questions and other sources, I seldom write

my experience as it happened but rather, I write the thought
that my experience nurtured. For example, many expressions
arise from my experience of dialysis in the early 1970s when
the procedures and equipment were primitive and many
friends suffered and died in anguish, with too much technology and not enough technology. Those years at the dialysis
unit are the words: "When the pain does not pass, hope is
the presence of care."

Phenomenology is research for living—our living. The
thematic questions arising from my written response to one
life are set in relief for my continued reflection by another
life. For example, Pauline's question, "How is self-pity
honorable?" remained to me an enigma until I read "I
Thought I Was Too Young" by David Cornelius. David's
description of his experience of illness helped me to articulate
themes of self-pity which lead through the experience of self-
pity to the experience of blessings. The question I had doubted
was the first step on a journey of hope with Pauline and David.

Reflecting on thematic difficulties in text helped me to
find questions that open up the way through the difficulty.
For example, "The Heart of Pity" is permeated with reflection
on a thematic impasse. One man wrote honestly that suffering
defeats the doctor (Why suffering? why defeat?); one man
spoke honestly in response, "Suffering does not defeat the
doctor" (Is this the absence of defeat or the refusal of defeat?).
I began to understand the impasse as dialectic when I
searched for the deep meaning of doctor there. The questions
I found helped me journey to the heart of pity.

Listening to interviewees respond to my writing helped
me to reflect on the adequacy of my expression in relation
to their experience. For example, in "Letting Go of the
Things," the chaplain helped me to reflect upon a thematic
description I had written which was inadequate to express
his experience of ministering to those who judged themselves
condemned, and therefore, condemned others like themselves;
but found God's mercy for themselves, and therefore, found
the other. He said that the relation of self to others is like
the relation of concave to convex in a glass bottle. There are
no others in Ivan's experience of condemnation. The glass

shatters. Ivan and others live in his experience of mercy. The thematic description for "Judgment to Mercy" was rewritten through this reflection.

Writing to understand is learning to let the themes "speak." For example, I had chosen to write the thematic statements in sentences. The sentence expressed the fullness of the themes of Pauline's experience. But the themes of Ivan's experience "expressed themselves" as A to B—terse and tentative, like Ivan's search.

Friendship

Learning to write and writing to learn requires a place. More than a desk and chair and bookshelves, a place is openness to the new researcher and the new researcher's question; a place is the friendship of teaching and learning. In the manner of friendship, Dr. Ted Aoki, then Chairman of the Department of Secondary Education, welcomed me. In the manner of friendship, he showed me much of what my research could be, though seldom speaking directly of it. In the manner of friendship, there was a place for silence, a place for question, a place for sharing: a place for me.

Learning to write and writing to learn requires a teacher. I learned to write with the help of the teacher, Dr. Max van Manen, who had walked the path of the research question in his writing. Unlike the writing of people I have not known, his writing is a part of his living conversation with me. If I could write like that. But my writing was the central text for dialogue with the teacher concerning the content and style of writing, the pathway of further interviewing, reading and writing—the research of writing. He taught me to write myself. For example, he asked me to write an example of what a chapter of research concerning illness might be like. I gave "On Pauline's Diary" as a possibility for research writing concerning the life of illness. He responded by giving me the writing of three phenomenologists: Heidegger, "On the Essence of Truth" and "The Origin of the Work of Art," Gadamer, "The Ontology of the Work of Art and Its Hermeneutic Significance," and Kierkegaard, *Fear and Trembling*.

These sources became the content and structure for the research writing of Chapter 6, "A Pathway for Theorizing." My writing, "On Pauline's Diary" entered into the tradition of research and became articulate for me as a way for continuing research through the guidance of a teacher. He had journeyed that way—he could show me the way. Yet always, he asked me to find the way by writing.

Learning to write and writing to learn is blessed by the fellowship of other students of the research question who are involved in formal study or are learning from life in whatever situation. For example, faculty and graduate students at the University of Alberta and I have shared our research concerns and writing. We have found a common purpose in our different pursuits. Our research springs from our daily life, for our daily life; we write because we want to give something good.

But how can I give something good unless I am with the One who is good? So prayer was an important part of my research. The thoughts I wrote are prayerful. Thought that comes from the heart of experience, which Gadamer calls pain, refers to the love that comes from God. As this love is the source of validity for our daily living, so it is the source of validity for research concerning our everyday lives. This one source of validity relates the researcher to the reader in dialogue: the researcher works to write the love that the reader lives, and the reader works to live the love that the researcher articulates.

> More things are wrought by prayer
> Than this world dreams of. Wherefore, let thy voice
> Rise like a fountain for me night and day.
> For what are men better than sheep or goats
> That nourish a blind life within the brain,
> If, knowing God, they lift not hands of prayer
> Both for themselves and those who call them friend?
> For so the whole round earth is every way
> Bound by gold chains about the feet of God.
>
> —Lord Tennyson[6]

NOTES

Chapter 3. The Question of Technology.

1. Samuel B. Chyatte, "To my fellow patients in the certain knowledge that life is more than survival," *Rehabilitation in Chronic Renal Failure*, Samuel B. Chyatte, ed. (Baltimore: Williams & Wilkins Co., 1979), Dedication page. Chyatte was a medical doctor on dialysis who died in 1979.

2. Cited in Heidegger, *The Question Concerning Technology and Other Essays*, (New York: Harper & Row, 1977), 59.

3. The full quotation is from Revelation 22: 16b, where Christ speaks, "I am the root and offspring of David, the bright morning star."

4. Bill Blackton, "We Were Pioneers," *NAPHT News*, (November 1979), 18. NAPHT is an acronym for National Association of Patients on Hemodialysis and Transplants.

5. Michael Olmsted, "Some Thoughts of a Kidney Disease Victim," *NAPHT News*, (January 1981), 7.

6. Carol Olson, "Technology's Children," (Class assignment for a course in phenomenological writing, taught by Professor Max van Manen, University of Alberta, January 1982).

7. Anonymous poem, cited by June Crowley, "Editor's Notebook," *NAPHT News*, (November 1977), 3.

8. Renee Fox and Judith Swazey, *The Courage to Fail: A Social View of Organ Transplants and Dialysis*, (Chicago: University of Chicago Press, 1978), 380. Representative critiques of modern medicine include: Ivan Illich, *Limits to Medicine: Medical Nemesis, the Expropriation of Health*, (London: Boyars, 1976), a critique of the "medicalization of life," for example, the hospitalization of birth,

179

death and the common cold, and the analgesic avoidance of pain and difficulty; R. Mendelsohn, *Confessions of a Medical Heretic*, (New York: Warner Books, 1979), an allegorical critique of medicine as a religious cult, with a plan for reform.

9. Cited in Stephen Karatheodoris, "Logos. An Analysis of the Social Achievement of Rationality," *Friends, Enemies, Strangers: Theorizing in Art, Science, and Everyday Life*, Alan Blum et al., eds. (Norwood, NJ: Ablex, 1979), 202–214.

10. Karatheodoris, 211.

11. Ernest Klein, *A Comprehensive Etymological Dictionary of the English Language*, (New York: Elsevier, 1971), 114.

12. Gordon McIntosh, Personal communication, September 1982.

13. Klein, 618.

14. Heraclitus, Fragment 50.

15. Heraclitus, Fragment 50.

16. Heraclitus, Fragment 63.

17. Victor Robinson, *White Caps: The Story of Nursing* (New York: Lippincott, 1946), 9–11, 13. Robinson describes hospitality and the development of hospitals from ancient times to 1946.

18. Heraclitus, Fragment 63.

Chapter 4. The Question of Understanding.

1. Martin Heidegger, *The Question Concerning Technology and Other Essays*, (New York: Harper & Row, 1977).

2. Edmund Husserl, "Phenomenology," *Realism and the Background of Phenomenology*, ed. R. Chisholm, (New York: The Free Press, 1960), 131.

3. Max van Manen, "An Experiment in Educational Theorizing: The Utrecht School," *Interchange*, 10 (1978–79), 49.

4. Max van Manen, "Linking Ways of Knowing With Ways of Being Practical," *Curriculum Inquiry*, 6 (1977), 213.

5. Maurice Merleau-Ponty, *The Visible and the Invisible*, (Evanston: Northwestern University Press, 1968), 134.

6. Hans-Georg Gadamer, *Truth and Method*, (New York: The Seabury Press, 1975), 266.

7. Martin Heidegger, *Being and Time*, (New York: Harper & Row, 1962), 49.

8. Max van Manen, "Edifying Theory: Serving the Good," *Theory Into Practice*, 21 (1982), 49.

9. Cited in Merleau-Ponty, 149.

10. W. H. Auden, *Sonnets from China XIV, W. H. Auden: Collected Poems*, E. Mendelson, ed. (London: Faber & Faber, 1976), 154.

11. Merleau-Ponty, 126.

12. Margaret Hunsberger, *The Encounter Between Reader and Text*, (Doctoral Dissertation, University of Alberta, 1983), 271.

13. Merleau-Ponty, 118.

14. Merleau-Ponty, 147.

15. Gadamer, 60.

16. Gadamer, 338.

17. Michael Polanyi, *The Tacit Dimension*, (New York: Doubleday, 1951).

18. Cited in Palmer, *Hermeneutics: Interpretation Theory in Schleiermacher, Dilthey, Heidegger and Gadamer*, (Evanston: Northwestern University Press, 1969), 133.

19. Cited in Gabriel Marcel, *Homo Viator: Introduction to a Metaphysics of Hope*, (Chicago: Henry Regnery Co., 1951), 28.

20. Emmanuel Levinas, *Totality and Infinity: An Essay on Exteriority*, A. Lingis, trans. (Pittsburgh: Duquesne University Press, 1969), for example, see 61.

21. Merleau-Ponty, 144.

22. Merleau-Ponty, 155.

23. Palmer, 186.

24. See Levinas, 1969.

Chapter 5. The Question of Theorizing.

1. Alan Blum, "Theorizing," *Understanding Everyday Life*, J. Douglas, ed. (Chicago: Aldine, 1970), 308.

2. Alan Blum, *Theorizing*, (London: Heinemann Educational Books, 1974), 20.

3. Blum, *Theorizing*, 132.

4. Blum, *Theorizing*, 34.

5. Blum, *Theorizing*, 74.

6. Blum, *Theorizing*, 77.

7. Talcott Parsons, *The Social System*, (New York: The Free Press, 1951).

8. Cited in S. Bloom, *The Doctor and His Patient: A Sociological Interpretation*, (New York: Russell Sage Foundation, 1963).

9. E. Freidson, "Client Control and Medical Practice," *American Journal of Sociology*, 65, (1960), 374–382.

10. Cited in H. Freeman, S. Levine, & L. Reeder, eds., *Handbook of Medical Sociology*, (Englewood Cliffs, N.J.: Prentice-Hall, 1972), 326.

11. Freidson, 374.

12. P. Berger and T. Luckman, *The Social Construction of Reality*, (New York: Penguin Books, 1966). 102; see also 105.

13. Ivan Illich, "Disabling Professions: Notes for a Lecture," *Contemporary Crises*, (1977), 361.

14. Norman Cousins, *Anatomy of an Illness as Perceived by the Patient: Reflections on Healing and Regeneration*, (New York: W.W. Norton, 1979), 160.

15. Cousins, 160.

16. R. Mendelsohn, *Confessions of a Medical Heretic*, (New York: Warner Books, 1979), 255–275

17. Mendelsohn, 260.

18. Mendelsohn, 260; see also 281.

19. Martin Heidegger, "The Question Concerning Technology" and "The Turning," *The Question Concerning Technology and Other Essays*, (New York: Harper & Row, 1977).

20. Emmanuel Levinas, *Otherwise Than Being or Beyond Essence*, A. Lingis, trans. (Boston: Nijhoff, 1981), 145.

21. B. Jager, "Theorizing, Journeying, Dwelling," *Phenomenological Psychology*, vol. 2 (1975), 235.

22. Heidegger, 1977, 28–33.

23. Jager, 253.

24. M. Heidegger, *Being and Time*, (New York: Harper & Row, 1962), for example, 42, 219–224.

25. George Steiner, *Heidegger*, (Glasgow: William Collins Sons & Co., 1978), 90.

26. Gabriel Marcel, *The Mystery of Being*, Vol. 1, (London: Harvard Press, 1950), 27, see also 29.

27. Steiner, 98.

Chapter 6. A Pathway for Theorizing.

1. Martin Heidegger, "On the Essence of Truth," *Basic Writings*, (New York: Harper & Row, 1977), 123. "Wonder at What Is: Language and Truthfulness" is based on this essay.

2. Heidegger, 124.

3. Heidegger, 124.

4. Heidegger, 125.

5. Heidegger, 127.

6. Heidegger, 135; see also 132.

7. Heidegger. 140.

8. Martin Buber, *Between Man and Man*, R. G. Smith, trans. (London: Collins Clear-Type Press, 1974), 54.

9. Heidegger, "The Origin of the Work of Art," *Basic Writings*, 173, 163.

10. H. G. Gadamer, "The Ontology of the Work of Art and Its Hermeneutical Significance," *Truth and Method*, (New York: Seabury Press, 1975), 113. The description of play as a clue to the origin of the work of art is based on this essay.

11. Gadamer, 99

12. Gadamer, 110.

13. Gadamer, 111.

14. Gadamer, 111.

15. Gadamer, 100.

16. See Heidegger, 163.

17. Gadamer, 102.

18. Richard Palmer, *Hermeneutics: Interpretation Theory in Schleiermacher, Dilthey, Heidegger and Gadamer*, (Evanston: Northwestern University Press, 1969), 169.

19. S. Kierkegaard, *Fear and Trembling/Repetition*, (Princeton, NJ: Princeton University Press, 1983).

20. Kierkegaard, 9.

21. Kierkegaard, 9.

22. Gen. 22:1–4, 6–13.

23. See Kierkegaard, 10–14.

24. Kierkegaard, 53.

25. Kierkegaard, 54.

26. Kierkegaard, 57.

27. Kierkegaard, 68.

28. Kierkegaard, 60.

29. Kierkegaard, 70.

30. Kierkegaard, 82.

31. Kierkegaard, 114.

32. Kierkegaard, 60.

33. Genesis 22:5.

34. Max van Manen, *Researching Lived Experience: Human Science for an Action Sensitive Pedagogy*, (London, Ont.: Althouse Press/Albany: SUNY Press, 1990).

35. Margaret Hunsberger, "The Encounter Between Reader and Text," Doctoral Dissertation, University of Alberta, 1983, 272.

36. David Hoy, *The Critical Circle*, (Berkeley: University of California Press, 1978), 49; see also Gadamer, 430.

Chapter 7. Ivan Ilyitch: One Against the Other Searches for the Other.

1. Leo Tolstoy, *The Death of Ivan Ilyitch*, C. Garnett, trans. (London: William Heineman, 1915).

2. G. Marcel, *Homo Viator: A Metaphysic of Hope*, E. Crawford, trans. (Chicago: Henry Regnery Co., 1951), 83.

3. Responses to *The Death of Ivan Ilyitch* were developed through dialogue with Rev. Dr. T. L. Leadbeater, retired Anglican minister and hospital chaplain, 27 October 1983.

4. Ernest Klein, *A Comprehensive Etymological Dictionary of the English Language*, (New York: Elsevier Pub. Co., 1971), 35.

5. Klein, 594.

6. Elsie Boulding, "Learning to Image the Future," *The Planning of Change*, Warren G. Bennis, ed. (3d ed.; N.Y.: Holt, Rinehart & Winston, 1976), 435.

7. Marcel, 502.

8. Victor Frankl, *The Will to Meaning: Foundations and Applications of Logotherapy*, (New York: World Pub. Co., 1969), 120.

9. Klein, 385.

10. Phillip Aries, *The Hour of Our Death*, H. Weaver, trans. (New York: Alfred A. Knopf, 1981), 566.

11. Aries, 565.

12. Martin Buber, *Between Man and Man*, R. G. Smith, trans. (London: Collins Clear-Type Press, 1974), 89.

13. Tolstoy, 51.

14. Aries, 564.

15. Bergsma and Thomasa, *Health Care: Its Psychosocial Dimensions*, (Pittsburgh: Duquesne University Press, 1982), for a sustained discussion of dis-ease in relation to disease.

16. Tolstoy, 56.

17. Gabriel Marcel, 46.

18. Maurice Merleau-Ponty, *Signs*, (Evanston: Northwestern University Press, 1964), 423, for a phenomenology of "time's synthesis" as the "action of a life which unfolds."

19. Emmanuel Levinas, *Totality and Infinity: An Essay on Exteriority*, A. Lingis, trans. (Pittsburgh: Duquesne University Press, 1969), 75.

20. Tolstoy, 51.

21. Bergsma & Thomasa, 165.

22. Tolstoy, 56.

23. Tolstoy, 67.

24. Tolstoy, 69.

25. John Keats, "After Dark Vapours," *The Physician in Literature*, Norman Cousins, ed. (Toronto: The Saunders Press, 1982), 384.

Chapter 8. Pauline Erickson: One with the Other.

1. Cited in Brian Erickson, "With All My Heart," *The Lutheran Standard*, 23 (1983), 12–16.

2. Klein, *A Comprehensive Etymological Dictionary of the English Language*, (New York: Elsevier Pub. Co., 1971), 810.

3. Paul Lindell, "Born to Trouble," World Mission Prayer League, Lutheran Missionary Fellowship, 1972, 25.

4. Acts 17:28.

5. Klein, 323.

6. J. H. van den Berg, *Psychology of the Sick Bed*, (Pittsburgh: Duquesne University Press, 1966).

7. Lindell, 31.

8. Gabriel Marcel, *The Mystery of Being*, Vol. 1, (London: The Harvard Press, 1950), 41.

9. Gabriel Marcel, *Homo Viator: A Metaphysics of Hope*, (Chicago: Henry Regnery Co., 1951), 32.

10. F. J. J. Buytendijk, *Pain*, (London: Hutchinson, 1961), 152.

11. Psalm 90:10.

12. G. Marcel, *Homo Viator*, 36.

13. M. Merleau-Ponty, *Signs*, (Evanston: Northwestern University Press, 1964), 15.

14. Cited in Marcel, *Homo Viator*, 28.

15. Erickson, 15.

16. Augustine, *Confessions of Saint Augustine*, (New York: Sheed & Ward, 1943), 68.

17. David Cornelius, "I Thought I Was Too Young," *Guideposts*, June 1984, 8, 9.

18. See Alfred, Lord Tennyson, "In Memoriam, A. H. H.," *Tennyson: Selected Poetry*, H. M. McLuhan, ed. (New York: Holt, Rinehart & Winston, 1966), 120, for a description of change as life from death, That men may rise on stepping-stones Of their dead selves to higher things.

19. Joni Eareckson Tada, (Televised Billy Graham Crusade, Los Angeles, California, September 1984).

20. John Milton, "When I Consider How My Light is Spent," *The Norton Anthology of English Lierature*, Vol. 1, M. H. Abrams, ed. (New York: W.W. Norton & Co., 1968), 1015.

21. Victor Frankl, *Man's Search for Meaning*, New York: Washington Square Press, 1963.

22. Martin Heidegger, *Being and Time*, J. Macquarrie & E. Robinson, trans. (New York: Harper & Row, 1962).

23. Buytendijk, 132, is writing generally about the experience of pain.

24. Matthew 28:20.

25. Percy Bysshe Shelley, "To a Skylark," *The Norton Anthology of English Literature*, Vol. 2, ed. M.H. Abrams, (New York: W.W. Norton & Co., 1968), 144.

Chapter 9. Dr. Rieux: One for the Other.

1. Albert Camus, *The Plague*, S. Gilbert, trans., Nobel Prize Library, Camus and Churchill, (New York: Alexis Gregory, 1971).

2. Camus, 8.

3. Emmanuel Levinas, *Otherwise Than Being or Beyond Essence*, A. Lingis, trans. (Boston: Nijhoff, 1981).

4. Camus, 29.

5. Eccles. 1:7,8a.

6. Cited in M. Greene, "Cognition, Consciousness and Curriculum," *Heightened Consciousness, Cultural Revolution, and Curriculum Theory*, Wm. Pinar, ed. (Berkeley: McCutchan, 1974), 74.

7. Responses to *The Plague* were developed through dialogue with a dialysis doctor, 28 September 1983.

8. Jer. 8:22.

9. Klein, *A Comprehensive Etymological Dictionary of the English Language*, (New York: Elsevier Pub. Co., 1971), 561.

10. Loren Eiseley, *The Star Thrower*, (London: Wildwood House, 1978), 169–185.

11. Eiseley, 172–173.

12. Eiseley, 182.

13. Eiseley, 184.

14. For an example of life-saving bone restoration research, see Hector F. DeLuca, "The Kidney as an Endocrine Organ Involved in the Function of Vitamin D," *The American Journal of Medicine*, 58, (1975), 39–56, for the biochemist's analysis; Donald S. Siverberg et al., *Canadian Medical Association Journal*, 112, (1975), 190–195, for the medical doctor's analysis; Arthur Olson, "The Olson's Three Miracles," *Reader's Digest*, (August 1976), 61–66, for Arthur's

description of his experience of rising from a wheelchair to walk, move with ease, and conduct his beloved music.

15. Aurelius Augustine, *Confessions of Saint Augustine*, F. J. Sheed, trans. (New York: Sheed & Ward, 1943), 68.

16. Albert Schweitzer, *Out of My Life and Thought*, C. T. Campion, trans. (New York: Henry Holt & Co., 1933), 279. The quotation in the thematic heading is found on the same page.

17. Schweitzer, 279.

18. Oliver Wendell Holmes, "Elsie Venner," In *The Physician in Literature*, Norman Cousins, ed. (Toronto: Holt, Rinehart & Winston, 1982), 224–230.

19. Holmes, 229.

20. Norman Cousins, *The Healing Heart*, (New York: W.W. Norton & Co., 1983), 128.

21. Schweitzer, 166.

22. Camus, 112.

23. Camus, 113.

24. Scribner, Belding G. "The Problem of Patient Selection for Treatment with an Artificial Kidney," Seattle, Washington, 1972, cited by Renee Fox & Judith Swazey, *The Courage to Fail*, (Chicago: University of Chicago Press, 1978), 202.

25. Emmanuel Levinas, *Otherwise Than Being or Beyond Essence*, A. Lingis, trans. (Boston: Nijhoff, 1981), 145.

Chapter 10. Florence Nightingale: One by the Other.

1. Martin Heidegger, *Being and Time*, J. Macquarrie and E. Robinson, trans. (New York: Harper & Row, 1962).

2. Cecil Woodham-Smith, *Florence Nightingale*, (Glasgow: William Collins & Sons Co., 1977), 185, biography; see also Florence Nightingale, *Notes on Nursing: What It Is and What It is Not*, (1869/1946 Montreal: Lippincott), instruction to student nurses. Biographical excerpt precedes instructional excerpt for each theme.

3. Responses to excerpts from *Notes on Nursing* were developed through dialogue with a dialysis nurse, 21 & 27 September 1984.

4. Ruth is a pseudonym. This example is reconstructed from interview notes.

5. Ted T. Aoki, To the concrete itself in studies in education: a response, "Re-thinking Education: Modes of Enquiry in the Human Sciences," Monograph 3, Dept. of Secondary Education, Faculty of Education, University of Alberta, 1981, 40.

6. John is a pseudonym. This example is reconstructed from interview notes.

7. Laura Copp, "The Spectrum of Suffering," *American Journal of Nursing*, 74, 3 (1974), 495.

8. Cited by Norman Cousins, *The Healing Heart*, (New York: W. W. Norton & Co., 1983), 149.

9. Elizabeth Lord, "My Crisis With Cancer," *American Journal of Nursing*, 74, 4 (1983), 649.

10. Lord, 649.

Chapter 11. Lord Tennyson: One without the Other.

1. Alfred, Lord Tennyson, "In Memoriam, A. H. H.," *Tennyson: Selected Poetry*, H. M. McLuhan, ed. (New York: Holt, Rinehart & Winston, 1966), 118–220.

2. Responses to excerpts from "In Memoriam, A. H. H." were developed through written dialogue with Mrs. Clara Olson, my mother: bereaved sister, daughter, wife and mother, 23 October 1982.

3. Klein, *A Comprehensive Etymological Dictionary of the English Language* (New York: Elsevier Pub. Co., 1971), 350.

4. Ibid.

5. van Manen, Personal communication, January 1985.

6. J. McRae, "In Flanders Fields," In *Canadian Anthology*, C. Klink, ed. (Toronto: Gage, 1966), 216.

7. Klein, 786.

8. Psalm 8:4.

9. I Sam. 12:23b. These words express King David's grief at the death of his infant son and his confidence of eternal life with God; see also Job 19:24.

Chapter 12. The Homecoming.

1. John 1:1–19.

2. Hebrews 13:15.

3. Luke 20:36; see also Romans 8:16.

Chapter 13. Epilogue.

1. Jim is a pseudonym.

2. Victor Frankl, *Man's Search for Meaning: An Introduction to Logotherapy* (New York: Washington Square Press, 1963), 65.

3. Jurritt Bergsma and David Thomasa, *Health Care: Its Psychosocial Dimensions*, (Pittsburgh: Duquesne University Press, 1982), 171.

4. Mike is a pseudonym.

5. Eccles. 11:1,2.

6. Cited in Mary Wilder Tileston, *Joy and Strength* (Minneapolis, Mn: World Wide Publications, 1901/1986), 351.

BIBLIOGRAPHY

Abrams, M., ed. *The Norton Anthology of English Literaure*. 2 Vols. New York: W.W. Norton & Co., 1968.

Aoki, T., ed. "Re-thinking Education: Modes of Enquiry in the Human Sciences." Monograph 3, Department of Secondary Education, Faculty of Education, University of Alberta, 1981.

Aoki, T. "Towards a Dialectic Between the Conceptual World and the Lived World: Transcending Instrumentalism in Curriculum Orientation." An invited paper for presentation at teacher education seminars, South Korea, 1982.

Aries, P. *The Hour of Our Death*. New York: Alfred A. Knopf, 1981.

Auden, W. H. *W. H. Auden Collected Poems*, ed. E. Mendelson. London: Faber & Faber, 1976.

Augustine, A. *Confessions of Saint Augustine*, trans. F. J. Sheed. New York: Sheed & Ward, 1943.

Bennis, W., ed. *The Planning of Change*. 3rd ed. New York: Holt, Rinehart & Winston, 1976.

Berger, P. and Luckman, T. *The Social Construction of Reality*. New York: Penguin Books, 1966.

Bergsma, J. and Thomasa, D. *Health Care: Its Psychosocial Dimensions*. Pittsburgh: Duquesne University Press, 1982.

Blackton, B. "We Were Pioneers," *NAPH News*, November 1979, 18, 19.

Bloom, S. *The Doctor and His Patient: A Sociological Interpretation*. New York: Russell Sage Foundation, 1963.

Blum, A. *Theorizing*. London: Heinemann Educational Books Ltd., 1974.

Blum, A. *Socrates: The Original and Its Images.* Boston: Routledge & Kegan Paul, 1978.

Blum, A. and McHugh, P., eds. *Friends, Enemies, Strangers: Theorizing in Art, Science, and Everyday Life.* Norwood, NJ.: Ablex, 1979.

Blum, A., McHugh, P., Raffel, S., Foss, D., eds. *On the Beginning of Social Inquiry.* London: Routledge & Kegan Paul, 1974.

Buber, M. *Between Man and Man,* trans. R. G. Smith. London: Collins Clear-Type Press, 1974.

Buytendijk, F. J. J. *Pain.* London: Hutchinson, 1961.

Camus, A. *The Plague,* trans. S. Gilbert. Nobel Prize Library, Camus and Churchill. New York: Alexis Gregory, 1971.

Chisholm, R., ed. *Realism and the Background of Phenomenology.* New York: The Free Press, 1960.

Chyatte, S., ed. *Rehabilitation in Chronic Renal Failure.* Baltimore: Williams & Wilkins Co., 1979.

Copp, L. "The Spectrum of Suffering," *The American Journal of Nursing,* 74, no. 3 (1974), 491–495.

Cornelius, D. "I Thought I Was Too Young," *Guideposts,* June 1984, 7–9.

Cousins, N., *Anatomy of an Illness as Perceived by the Patient: Reflections on Healing and Regeneration.* New York: W.W. Norton, 1979.

Cousins, N., ed. *The Physician in Literature.* Toronto: Holt, Rinehart & Winston, 1982.

Cousins, N. *The Healing Heart.* New York: W.W. Norton, 1983.

Crowley, J., ed. "Editor's Notebook," *NAPHT News,* November 1977, 3.

Daabous, G. "Good-bye, My Village." Mississauga, Ont.: World Vision Int., 1984.

Daly, J. "Merleau-Ponty's Concept of Phenomenology," *Philosophical Studies,* 16 (1967), 137–164.

De Luca, H.F. "The Kidney as an Endocrine Organ Involved in the Function of Vitamin D," *The American Journal of Medicine,* 58 (1975), 39–56.

Douglas, J., ed. *Understanding Everyday Life.* Chicago: Aldine, 1970.

Eareckson Tada, J. Televised communication, World Wide Pictures, Inc., September 1984.

Eiseley, L. *The Star Thrower.* London: Wildwood House, 1978.

Eisner, E. and Vallance, E., eds. *Conflicting Conceptions of Curriculum.* Berkeley: McCutchan, 1974.

Erickson, B. "With All My Heart," *The Lutheran Standard*, 23 (1983), 12–15.

Field, P. A. "A Phenomenological Look at Giving an Injection," *Journal of Advanced Nursing*, 6 (1981), 291–296.

Fox, R. and Swazey, J. *The Courage to Fail: A Social View of Organ Transplants and Dialysis.* 2d ed., rev. Chicago: University of Chicago Press, 1978.

Frankl, V. *Man's Search for Meaning: An Introduction to Logotherapy.* New York: Washington Square Press, 1963.

Frankl, V. *The Will to Meaning: Foundations and Applications of Logotherapy.* New York: World, 1969.

Freeman, H., Levine, S. and Reeder, L., eds. *Handbook of Medical Sociology.* Englewood Cliffs, NJ: Prentice-Hall, 1972.

Freidson, E. "Client Control and Medical Practice," *American Journal of Sociology*, 65 (1960), 374–382.

Gadamer, H. G. *Truth and Method.* New York: The Seabury Press, 1975.

Heidegger, M. *Being and Time.* New York: Harper & Row, 1962.

Heidegger, M. *Poetry, Language, Thought.* New York: Harper & Row, 1971.

Heidegger, M. *Basic Writings.* New York: Harper & Row, 1977.

Heidegger, M. *The Question Concerning Technology and Other Essays.* New York: Harper & Row, 1977.

Highet, G. *The Art of Teaching.* Toronto: Random House, 1950.

Hoy, D. *The Critical Circle.* Berkeley: University of California Press, 1978.

Hunsberger, M. "The Encounter Between Reader and Text." Doctoral Dissertation, University of Alberta, 1983.

Illich, I. *Limits to Medicine: Medical Nemesis, the Expropriation of Health.* London: Boyars, 1976.

Illich, I. "Disabling Professions: Notes for a Lecture," *Contemporary Crises,* 1 (1977), 359–370.

Jager, B. "Theorizing, Journeying, Dwelling," *Phenomenological Psychology.* Vol. 2. Pittsburgh: Duquesne University Press, 1975.

Kelpin, V. "Birthing Pain," *Phenomenology + Pedagogy,* 2 (1984), 178–190.

Kierkegaard, S. *Fear and Trembling/Repetition,* eds. and trans. H. Hong and E. Hong. Princeton, NJ.: Princeton University Press, 1983.

Klein, E. *A Comprehensive Etymological Dictionary of the English Language.* New York: Elsevier, 1971.

Klink, C., ed. *Canadian Anthology.* Toronto: Gage, 1966.

Kubler-Ross, E. *On Death and Dying.* New York: Macmillan, 1970.

Kwant, R. *Encounter.* Pittsburgh: Duquesne University Press, 1965.

Leadbeater, T. L., Reverend Dr. (Anglican minister, hospital and nursing home chaplain). Interview. 27 Oct. 1983.

Levinas, E. *Totality and Infinity: An Essay on Exteriority,* trans. A. Lingis. Pittsburgh: Duquesne University Press, 1969.

Levinas, E. *Otherwise Than Being or Beyond Essence,* trans. A. Lingis. Boston: Martinus Nijhoff, 1981.

Levinas, E. *Ethics and Infinity.* Pittsburgh: Duquesne University Press, 1985.

Lindell, P. "Born to Trouble." World Mission Prayer League, Lutheran Missionary Fellowship, 1972.

Lord, E. "My Crisis With Cancer," *American Journal of Nursing,* 74 (1983), 647–649.

McIntosh, G. Personal communication, Dept. of Educational Administration, University of Alberta, September 1982.

Marcel, G. *The Mystery of Being*. Vol. 1. London: The Harvell Press, 1950.

Marcel, G. *Homo Viator: A Metaphysic of Hope*, trans. E. Crawford. Chicago: Henry Regnery, 1951.

Mendelsohn, R. *Confessions of a Medical Heretic*. New York: Warner Books, 1979.

Merleau-Ponty, M. *Signs*. Evanston: Northwestern University Press, 1964.

Merleau-Ponty, M. *The Primacy of Perception*. Evanston: Northwestern University Press, 1964.

Merleau-Ponty, M. *The Visible and the Invisible*, trans. A. Lingis. Evanston: Northwestern University Press, 1968.

Nightingale, F. *Notes on Nursing: What It Is and What It is Not*. Montreal: Lippincott, 1869/1946.

Olmsted, M. "Some Thoughts of a Kidney Disease Victim," *NAPHT News*, January 1981, 7, 8.

Olson, A. "The Olson's Three Miracles," as told to Sidney Katz, *Reader's Digest*, August 1976, 61–66.

Olson, C. "Technology's Children," Class assignment, January 1982.

Olson, Clara. Interview, 23 Oct. 1983.

Palmer, R. *Hermeneutics: Interpretation Theory in Schleiermacher, Dilthey, Heidegger and Gadamer*. Evanston: Northwestern University Press, 1969.

Parsons, T. *The Social System*. New York: The Free Press, 1951.

Pinar, William. "Life History and Educational Experience," *Journal of Curriculum Theorizing*, (September 1980), 159–212.

Plato, "Meno," *Protagoras and Meno*, trans. W. K. C. Guthrie. New York: Penguin Books, 1979.

Polanyi, M. *The Tacit Dimension*. New York: Doubleday, 1967.

Ricoeur, P. *Essays on Biblical Interpretation*. Philadelphia: Fortress Press, 1980.

Robinson, B. *White Caps: The Story of Nursing.* New York: Lippincott, 1946.

Schweitzer, A. *Out of My Life and Thought,* trans. C. T. Campion. New York: Henry Holt, 1933.

Silverberg, D., et al. "Effect of 1,25-dihydroxy-cholecalciferol in Renal Osteodystrophy," *Canadian Medical Association Journal,* 112 (1979), 190–195.

Smith, D. "Learning to Live in the Home of Language: Hearing the Pedagogic Voice as Poetic," *Phenomenology + Pedagogy,* 1 no. 1 (1983), 29–35.

Spiegelberg, H. *The Phenomenological Movement: A Historical Introduction.* 2 Vols. The Hague: Nijhoff, 1960.

Steiner, G. *Heidegger.* Glasgow: William Collins Sons, 1978.

Suransky, V. "Phenomenology: An Alternative Research Paradigm and a Force for Social Change," *Journal of the British Society for Phenomenology,* 11 (1980), 163–178.

Tennyson, A. *Tennyson: Selected Poetry,* ed. H. M. McLuhan. New York: Holt, Rinehart & Winston, 1850/1966.

Tileston, Mary Wilder. *Joy and Strength.* Minneapolis, Mn: World Wide Publications, 1901/1986.

Tolstoy, L. *The Death of Ivan Ilyitch,* trans. C. Garnett. London: William Heineman, 1915.

Van den Berg, J. H. *Psychology of the Sick Bed.* Pittsburgh: Duquesne University Press, 1966.

Van den Berg, J.H. *The Changing Nature of Man.* New York: Dell, 1975.

Van Manen, M. "Linking Ways of Knowing With Ways of Being Practical," *Curriculum Inquiry,* 6 (1977), 205–288.

Van Manen, M. "An Experiment in Educational Theorizing: The Utrecht School," *Interchange,* 10 (1978–1979), 48–66.

Van Manen, M. "Edifying Theory: Serving the Good," *Theory Into Practice,* 21, (1982), 44, 49.

Van Manen, M. "Phenomenological Pedagogy," *Curriculum Inquiry,* 12 (1982), 283–299.

Van Manen, M., ed. "Teaching and Doing Phenomenology," *Phenomenology + Pedagogy*, 2 no. 1 (1984), 1–72.

Van Manen, M. "Action Research as Theory of the Unique: From Pedagogic Thoughtfulness to Pedagogic Tactfulness." In *The Action Research Reader*, Deakin University Press, 1987.

Van Manen, M. *Researching Lived Experience: Human Science for an Action Sensitive Pedagogy*. Albany: SUNY Press; London, Ont.: Althouse Press, 1990.

Walker, H.A. "How and Why I Write: An Interview With Elie Wiesel," *Journal of Education*, (Spring 1980), 57–63.

Woodham-Smith, C. *Florence Nightingale*. Glasgow: William Collins & Sons, 1977.

Zaner, R. *The Problem of Embodiment: Some Contributions to a Phenomenology of the Body*. The Hague: Nijhoff, 1971.

INDEX